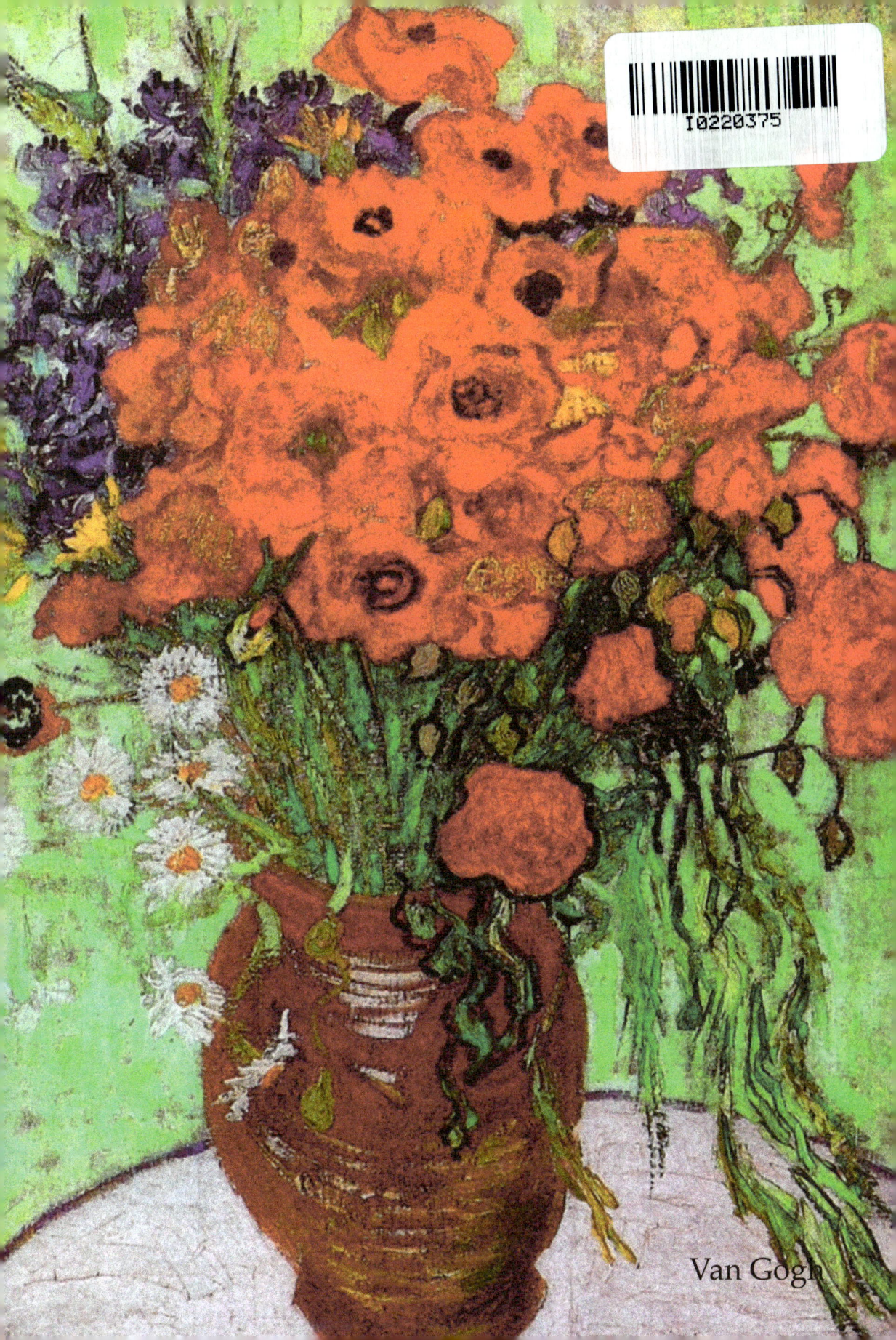

Van Gogh

A Dovetale Press Adaptation

The Garden Party & The Doll's House

Katherine Mansfield

Adaptation by
Dr Gillian Claridge
Dr B. Sally Rimkeit

Art by
Paul Cézanne
Gustav Klimt
August Macke
Amedeo Modigliani
Vincent Van Gogh

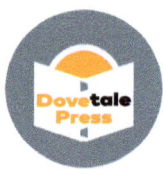

A Dovetale Press Adaptation
The Garden Party & The Doll's House
Katherine Mansfield

Adapted by Dr Gillian Claridge and Dr B. Sally Rimkeit
Copyright 2016 © Gillian Claridge and B. Sally Rimkeit

All original materials in Public Domain
Illustrations from Awesome Art
Original text from Project Gutenberg
Photograph of Katherine Mansfield from the Alexander Turnbull Library, Wellington, New Zealand

This edition published by Dovetale Press 2016

National Library of New Zealand Cataloguing-in-Publication Data:
Claridge, Gillian
A Dovetale Press Adaptation The Garden Party & The Doll's House Katherine Mansfield / Gillian Claridge and B. Sally Rimkeit; original text from Project Gutenberg
ISBN 978-0-473-37291-0
I. Rimkeit, Sally, 1958- II. Mansfield, Katherine, 1888-1923. Garden party
III. Mansfield, Katherine, 1888-1923. Doll's House. IV. Title.
NZ823.3—dc 23

Comments and questions, please email: editor@dovetalepress.com

All titles in this Dovetale Press series are carefully constructed to enhance readability. Our other titles are
A Dovetale Books Adaptation of A Christmas Carol by Charles Dickens ISBN 978-0-473-37294-1
A Dovetale Press Adaptation of Little Women by Louisa May Alcott ISBN 978-0-473-37295-8
A Dovetale Press Adaptation of Sherlock Holmes: The Adventure of the Blue Carbuncle by Arthur Conan Doyle ISBN 978-0-473-37293-4
A Dovetale Press Selection: Poetry for the Restless Heart
ISBN 978-0-473-37292-7

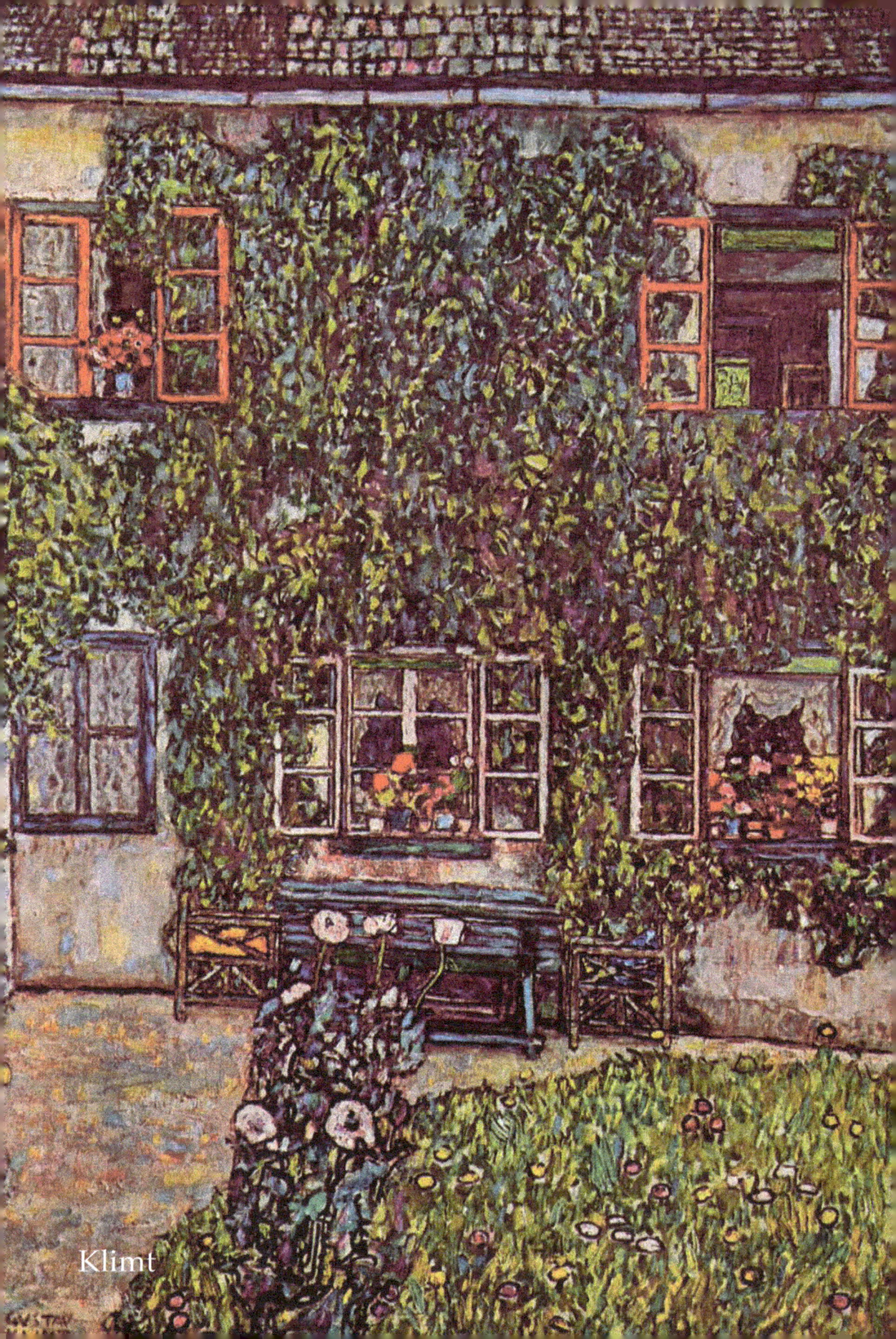

CONTENTS

THE GARDEN PARTY	6
Cast of Characters	7
Précis of story	37
THE DOLL'S HOUSE	38
Cast of characters	39
Précis of story	62
About Katherine Mansfield	63

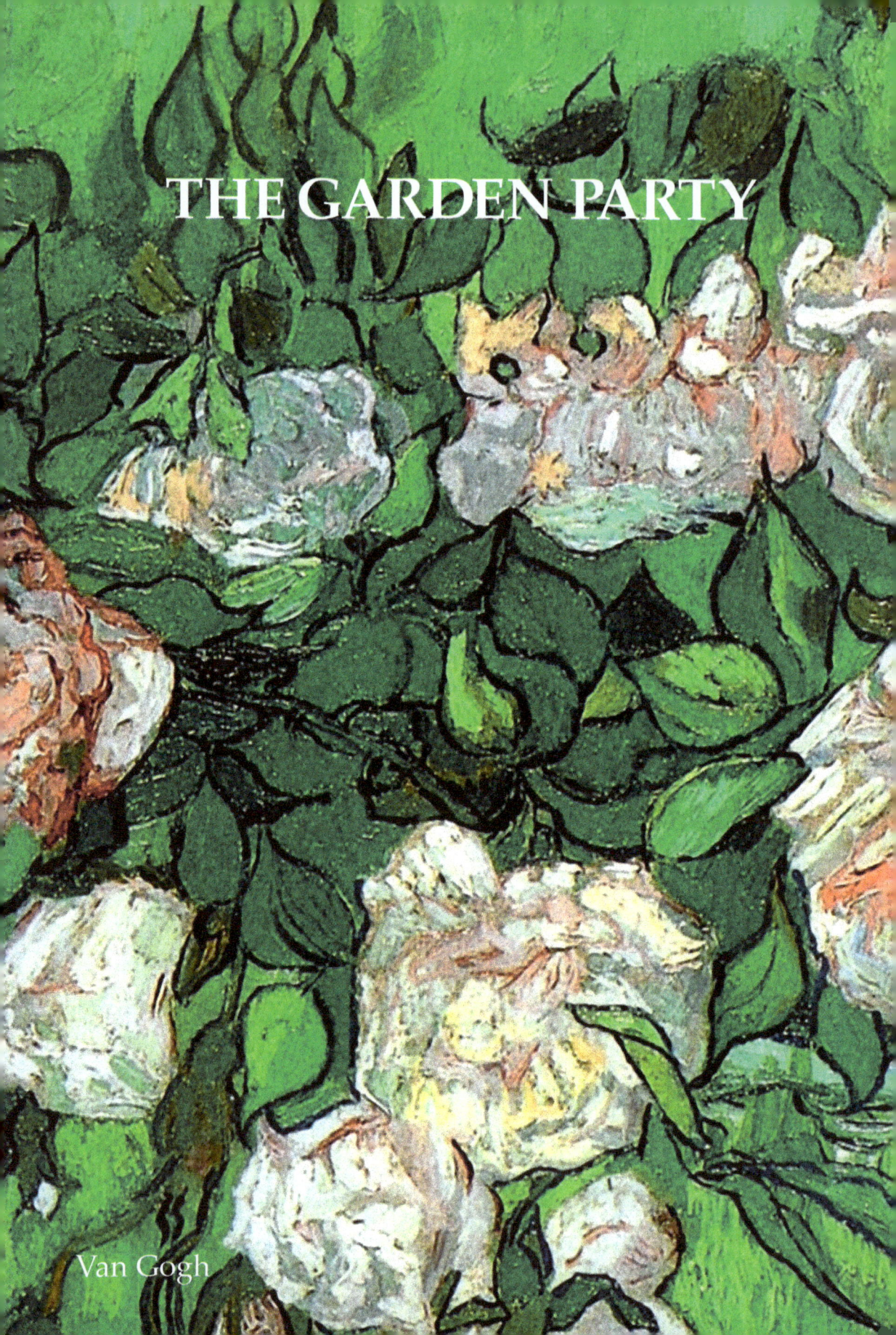

CAST OF CHARACTERS

Mr and Mrs Sheridan, rich people who are holding a garden party

Laura Sheridan, their daughter
Jose Sheridan, their daughter
Laurie Sheridan, their son

The tall man who comes to put up the marquee

Cook, the Sheridans' cook
Sadie, the Sheridans' maid
Godber's man, who delivers the cream puffs

Mr Scott, who is killed in an accident with a cart
Em, his widow
Em's sister, a little woman dressed in black

THE GARDEN PARTY

And after all the weather was ideal. The Sheridans could not have had a more perfect day for a garden party if they had ordered it. Windless, warm, the sky without a cloud.

As for the roses, you could not help feeling they understood that roses are the only flowers that impress people at garden parties. The green bushes bowed down as though they had been visited by archangels.

Breakfast was not yet over before the men came to put up the marquee.

Mrs Sheridan said to her daughter: "You'll have to tell them where to put it up, Laura. You're the artistic one."

"Good morning," she said to the men, copying her mother's voice. But that sounded so fearfully affected that she was ashamed and stammered like a little girl, "Oh – er – have you come – is it about the marquee?"

"That's right, miss," said the tallest of the men, and smiled down at her. "That's about it. We'll put it in front of those trees."

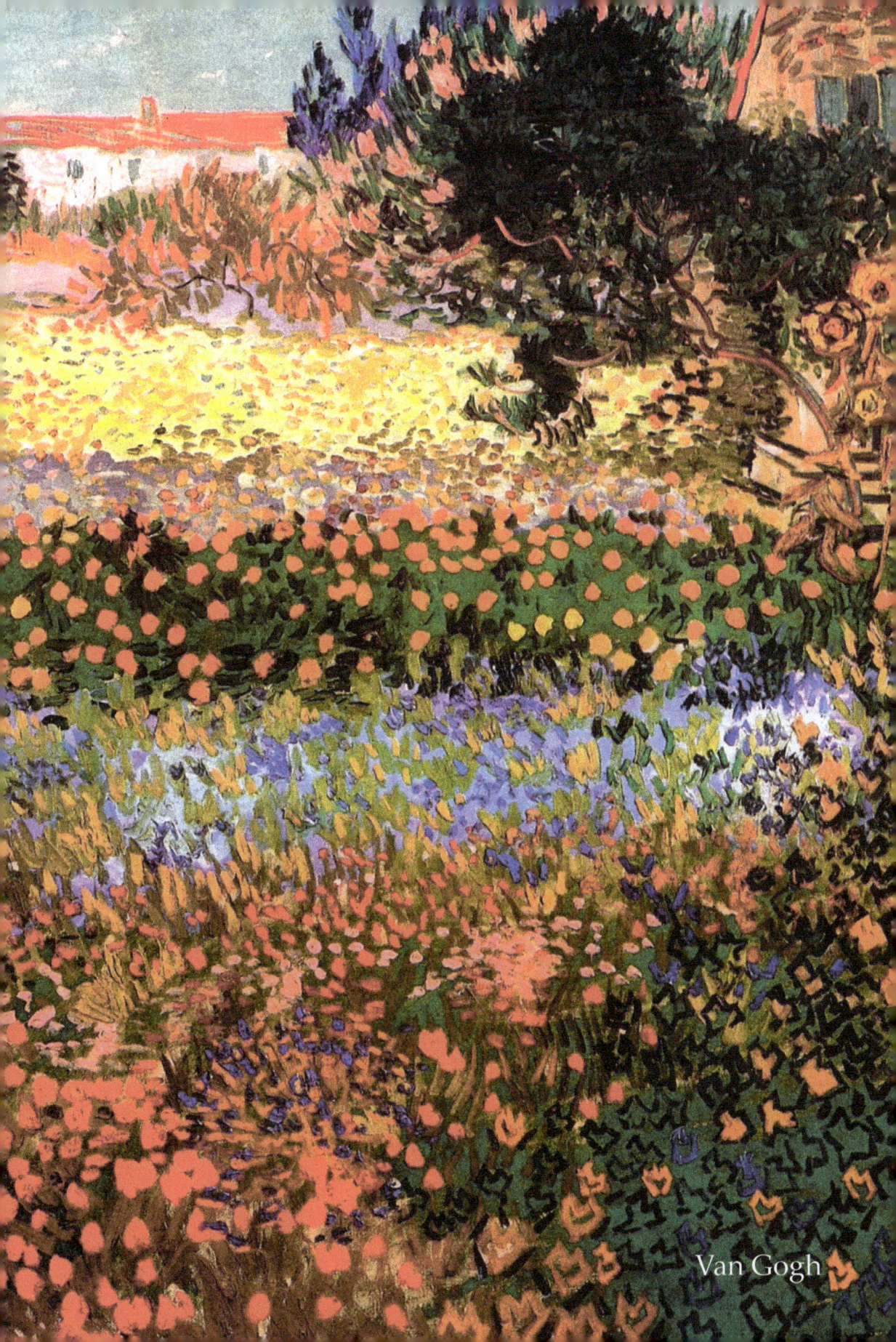

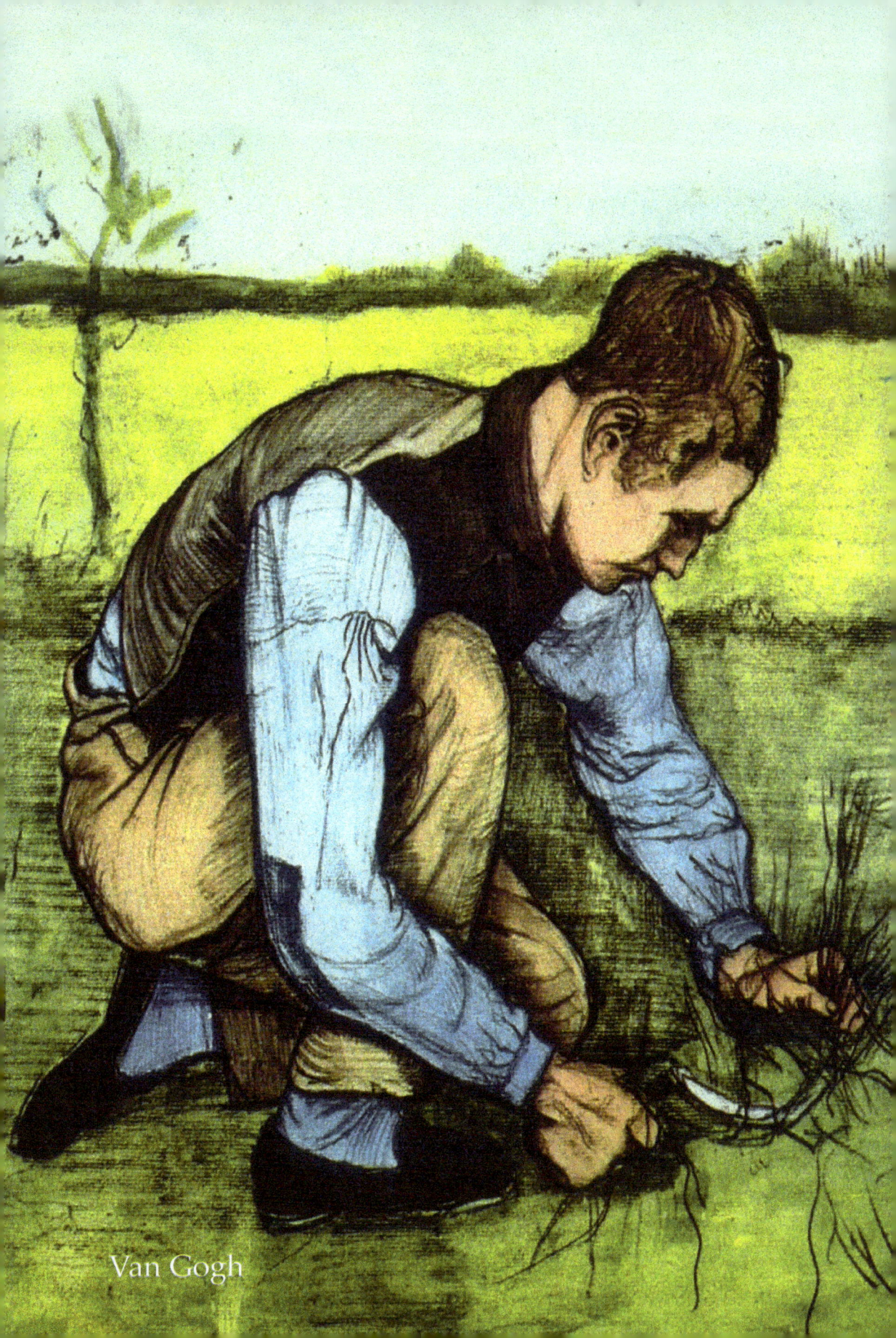

THE GARDEN PARTY

The men shouldered their staves and made for the lawn in front of the karaka trees.

Only the tall fellow was left. He bent down, pinched a sprig of lavender, put his thumb and forefinger to his nose and snuffed up the smell. When Laura saw that gesture, she forgot all about the marquee in her wonder at him caring for things like that – caring for the smell of lavender.

How many men that she knew would have done such a thing? Oh, how extraordinarily nice workmen were, she thought. Why couldn't she have workmen for her friends rather than the silly boys she danced with and who came to Sunday night supper? She would get on much better with men like these.

"Laura, Laura, where are you? Telephone, Laura!" a voice cried from the house.

"Coming!" Away she skimmed, over the lawn, up the path, up the steps, across the veranda, and into the porch.

In the hall Laura's father and her brother Laurie were brushing their hats ready to go to the office. Suddenly Laura couldn't stop herself. She ran at Laurie and gave him a small, quick squeeze. "Oh, I do love parties, don't you?" she gasped.

Sadie the maid asked Mrs Sheridan: "If you please, m'm, Cook says have you got the flags for the sandwiches?"

"The flags for the sandwiches, Sadie?" echoed Mrs Sheridan dreamily, "Let me see." And the children knew by her face that she hadn't got them. She said to Sadie firmly, "Tell Cook I'll let her have them in ten minutes."

The flags were finished at last, and Laura took them off to the kitchen. She found her sister Jose there talking to the cook.

"I have never seen such exquisite sandwiches," said Jose's rapturous voice. "How many kinds did you say there were, Cook? Fifteen?"

"Fifteen, Miss Jose."

THE GARDEN PARTY

"Well, Cook, I congratulate you."

Cook swept up crusts with the long sandwich knife, and smiled broadly.

"Godber's has come," announced Sadie, issuing out of the pantry. She had seen the man pass the window.

That meant the cream puffs had come. Godber's were famous for their cream puffs. Nobody ever thought of making them at home.

"Bring them in and put them on the table, my girl," ordered Cook.

Sadie brought them in and went back to the door. Of course Laura and Jose were far too grown-up to really care about such things.

All the same, they couldn't help agreeing that the puffs looked very attractive. Very. Cook began arranging them, shaking off the extra icing sugar.

"Have one each, my dears," Cook said in her comfortable voice. "Yer ma won't know."

Oh, impossible. Fancy, cream puffs so soon after breakfast. The very idea made one shudder. All the same, two minutes later Jose and Laura were licking their fingers with that absorbed inward look that only comes from whipped cream.

"Let's go into the garden, out by the back way," suggested Laura.

But the back door was blocked by Cook, Sadie and Godber's man. Something had happened.

"Tuk-tuk-tuk," clucked Cook like an agitated hen. Sadie had her hand clapped to her cheek as though she had toothache. Only Godber's man seemed to be enjoying himself; it was his story.

"What's the matter? What's happened?"

"There's been a horrible accident," said Cook. "A man killed."

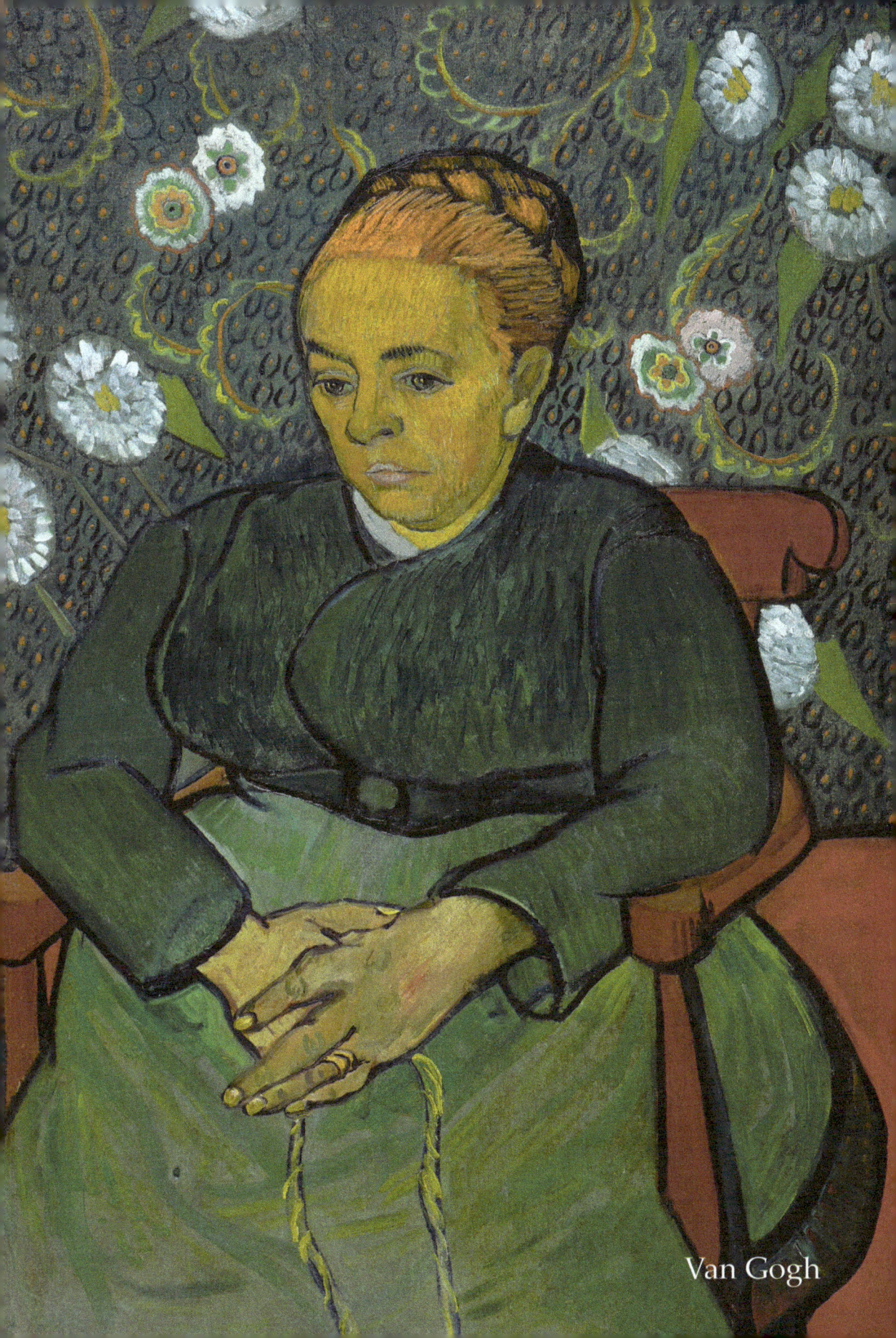

Godber's man said: "Know those little cottages just below here, miss? Well, there's a young chap living there, name of Scott, a carter. His horse shied at a traction-engine, corner of Hawke Street this morning, and he was thrown out on the back of his head. Killed."

"Dead!" Laura stared at Godber's man.

"Yes. He's left a wife and five little ones."

"Jose, come here." Laura caught hold of her sister's sleeve and dragged her through the kitchen to the other side of the green baize door. There she paused and leaned against it. "Jose!" she said, horrified, "however are we going to stop everything?"

"Stop everything, Laura!" cried Jose in astonishment. "What do you mean?"

"Stop the garden party, of course." Why did Jose pretend?

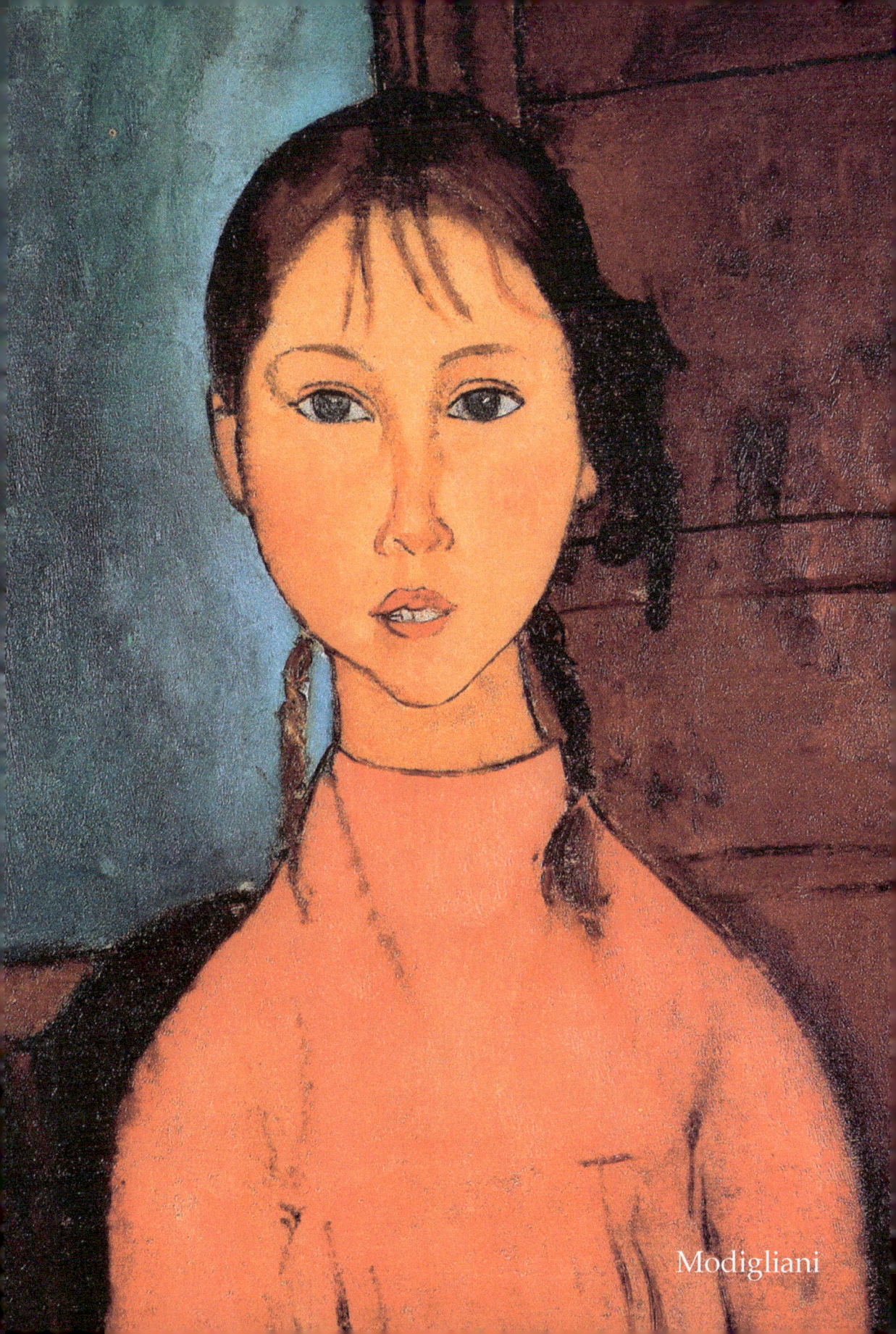

But Jose was still more amazed. "Stop the garden party? My dear Laura, don't be so absurd. Of course we can't do anything of the kind."

"But we can't possibly have a garden party with a man dead just outside the front gate," said Laura.

Of course it was not just outside the front gate although, true, the little cottages were far too near the Sheridans' house. They were little, mean dwellings painted a chocolate brown. In the garden patches there was nothing but cabbage stalks, sick hens and tomato cans. The very smoke coming out of their chimneys was poverty-stricken. Little rags and shreds of smoke, so unlike the great silvery plumes that uncurled from the Sheridans' chimneys.

"And just think of what the band would sound like to that poor woman," said Laura.

"Oh, Laura!" Jose began to be annoyed. "You won't bring a drunken workman back to life by being sentimental," she said softly.

Laura turned furiously on Jose. "Drunk! Who said he was drunk? I'm going straight up to tell mother."

She went up to Mother's room. Mrs Sheridan was trying on a new hat.

"Mother, a man's been killed," began Laura.

"Not in the garden?" interrupted her mother.

"No, no!"

"Oh, what a fright you gave me!" Mrs Sheridan sighed with relief.

"But listen, Mother," said Laura.

Breathless, half-choking, Laura told the dreadful story. "Of course, we can't have our party, can we?" she pleaded. "The band and everybody arriving. They'd hear us. Mother, they're nearly neighbours!"

To Laura's astonishment her mother behaved just like Jose; she refused to take Laura seriously.

"Mother, isn't it terribly heartless of us?" said Laura.

"Darling!" Mrs Sheridan got up and came over to her, carrying the new hat. Before Laura could stop her she had popped it on.

"My child!" said her mother, "this hat is yours. It's too young for me."

"But, Mother," Laura began again.

This time Mrs Sheridan lost patience just as Jose had done.

"You are being very absurd, Laura," she said coldly. "People like that don't expect sacrifices from us."

"I don't understand," said Laura, and she walked quickly out of the room into her own bedroom.

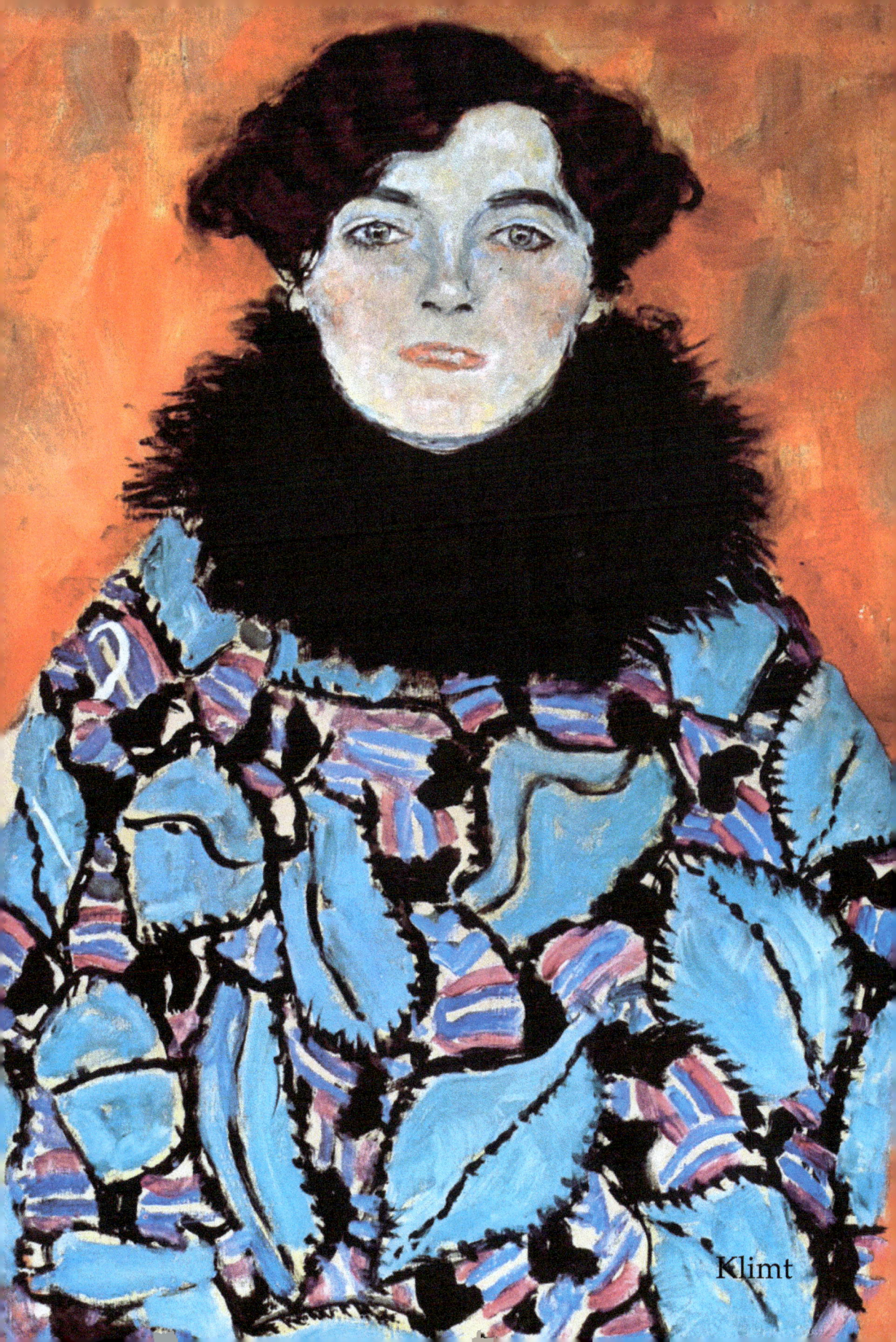

There, quite by chance, the first thing Laura saw was herself in the mirror, in her black hat trimmed with gold daisies, and a long black velvet ribbon. Never had she imagined she could look so charming.

Is Mother right? she thought. Am I absurd to want to cancel the garden party?

Laurie came home for the party, and at the sight of him, Laura remembered the accident again. She wanted to tell him.

"Laurie!" she said.

"Hallo!" He was half-way upstairs, but when he turned round and saw Laura he suddenly puffed out his cheeks and goggled his eyes at her. "My word, Laura! You do look stunning," said Laurie. "What an absolutely topping hat!"

Laura said faintly "Is it?" and smiled up at Laurie, and didn't tell him after all.

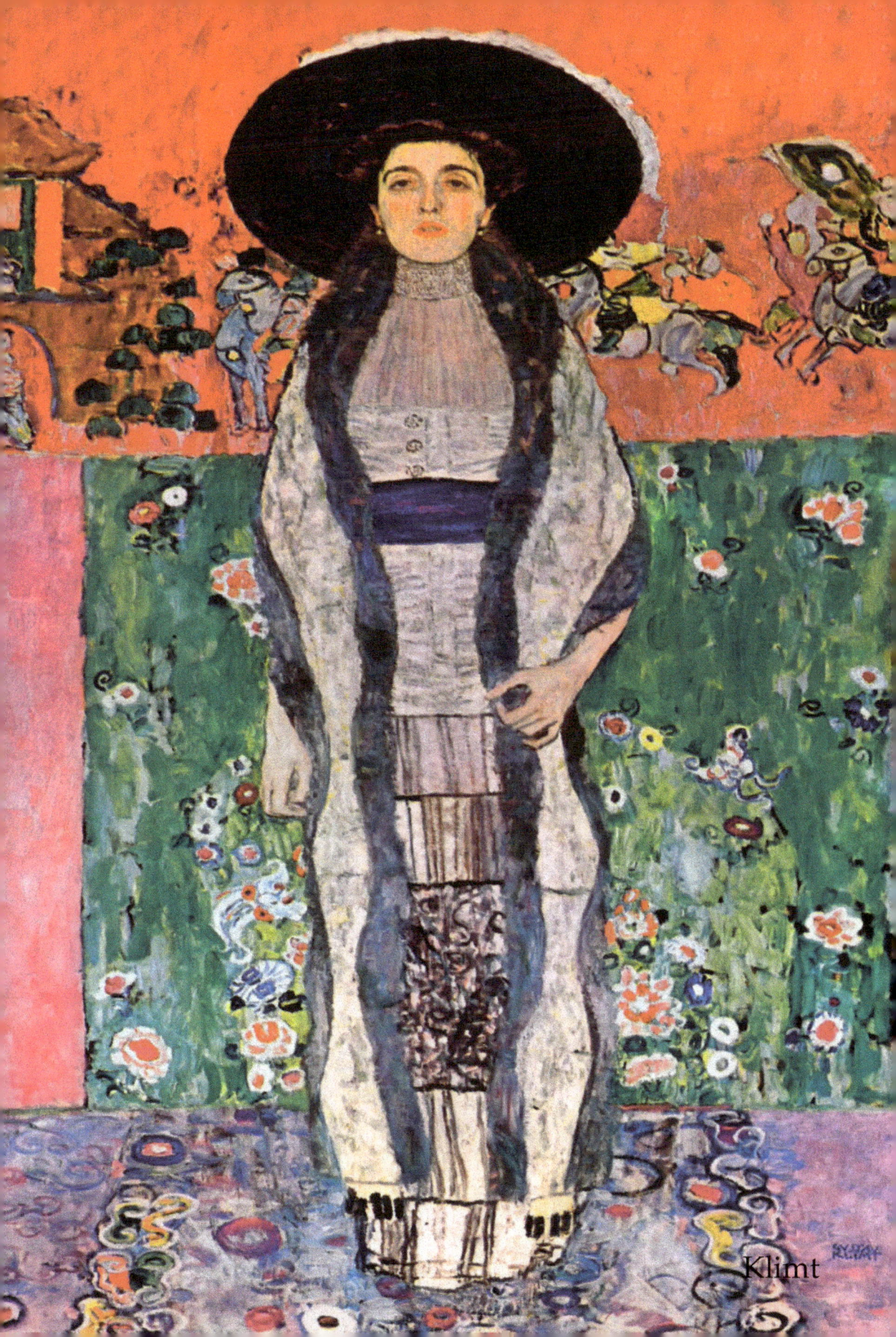

Soon after that, garden party guests began coming in streams. The band struck up. The hired waiters ran from the house to the marquee. Wherever you looked there were couples strolling, bending to the flowers, greeting, moving on over the lawn. They were like bright birds that had alighted in the Sheridans' garden for this one afternoon, on their way to – where?

And the perfect afternoon slowly ripened, slowly faded, slowly its petals closed.

"Never a more delightful garden party…"
"The greatest success…" "Quite the most…"

Laura helped her mother with the good-byes. They stood side by side in the porch till it was all over.

"All over, all over, thank heaven," said Mrs Sheridan. "Round up the others, Laura. Let's go and have some fresh coffee. I'm exhausted. Yes, it's been very successful."

And then the Sheridans sat down in the deserted marquee.

Mr Sheridan said: "I suppose you didn't hear of a beastly accident that happened to-day?"

"My dear," said Mrs Sheridan, holding up her hand, "We did. It nearly ruined the party. Laura insisted we should put it off."

"Oh, Mother!" Laura didn't want to be teased about it.

"It was a horrible affair all the same," said Mr Sheridan. "The chap was married too. Lived just below in the lane, and leaves a wife and half a dozen kiddies, so they say."

An awkward little silence fell. Mrs Sheridan fidgeted with her cup. Really, it was very tactless of Mr Sheridan…

Suddenly Mrs Sheridan looked up. There on the table were all those sandwiches, cakes, puffs, all uneaten, all going to be wasted. She had one of her brilliant ideas.

"I know," she said. "Let's make up a basket. Let's send that poor creature who's just lost her husband some of this perfectly good food. At any rate, it will be the greatest treat for the children."

"But, Mother, do you really think it's a good idea?" said Laura. Would the poor woman really like that? To take scraps from their party. How curious, Laura seemed to be different from them all.

"Of course! What's the matter with you to-day? An hour or two ago you were insisting on us being sympathetic, and now – " said Mother.

Oh well! Laura ran for the basket. It was filled, it was heaped by her mother.

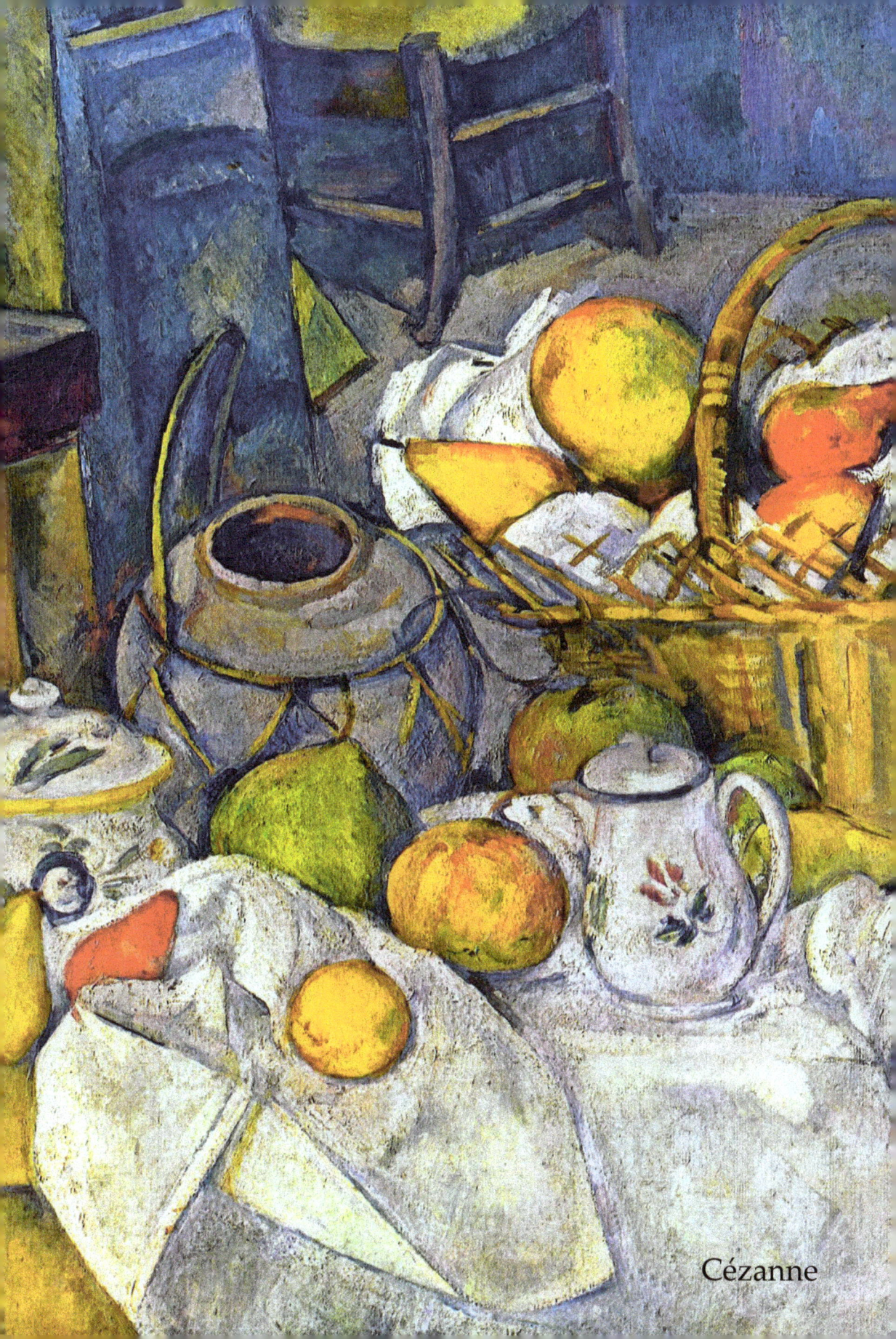

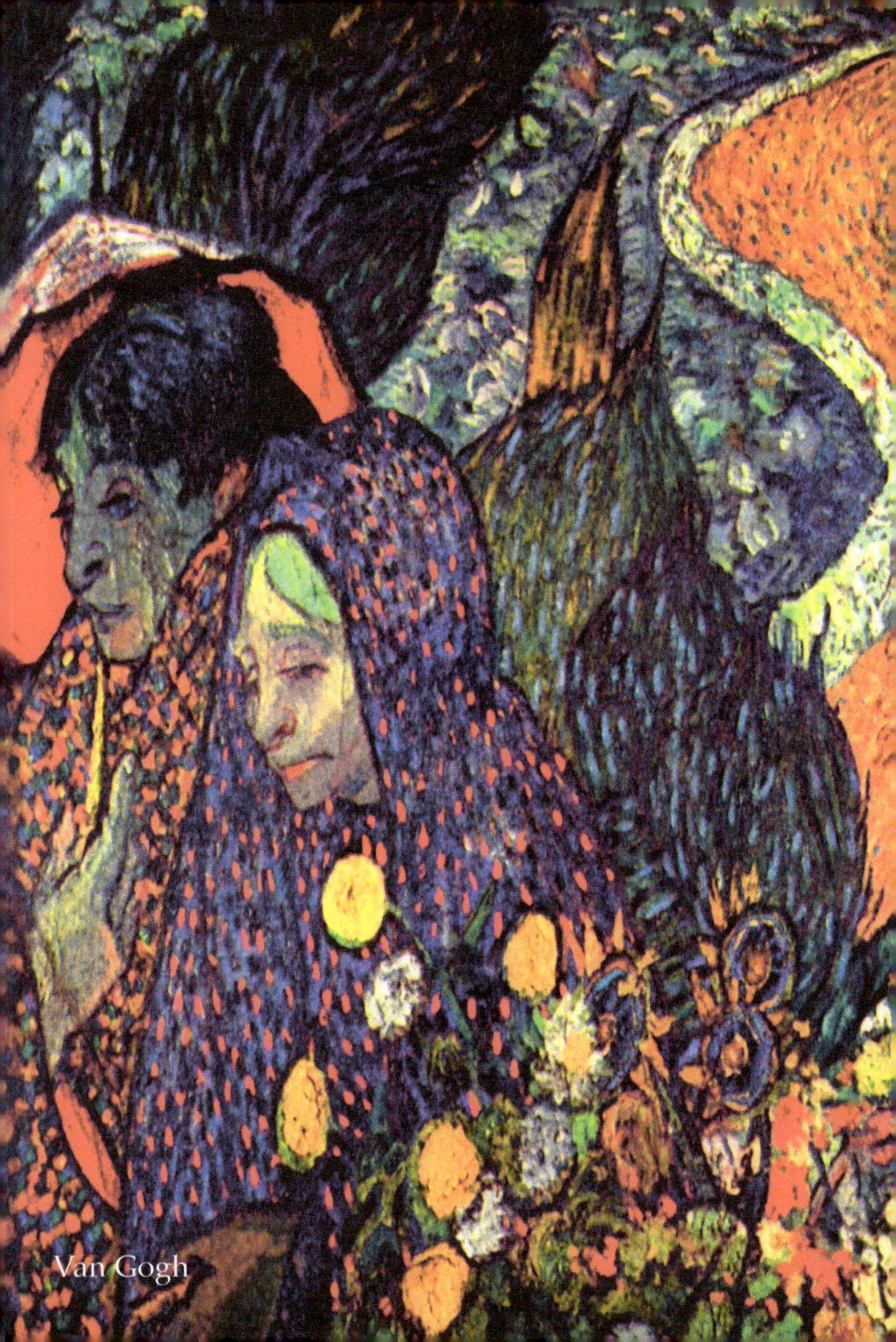
Van Gogh

It was just growing dusky as Laura shut their garden gates. A big dog ran by like a shadow. How quiet it seemed after the afternoon.

Here she was going down the hill to somewhere where a man lay dead, and she couldn't realize it. Why couldn't she?

And it seemed to her that kisses, voices, tinkling spoons, laughter, the smell of crushed grass were somehow inside her. She had no room for anything else. All she thought was, "Yes, it was the most successful party."

Now the broad road was crossed. The lane began, smoky and dark. Women in shawls and men's tweed caps hurried by. A low hum came from the mean little cottages.

Laura bent her head and hurried on. How her frock shone! And the big hat with the velvet streamer – if only it was another hat! It was a mistake to have come; should she go back even now?

No, too late. This was the house. It must be.

Laura was terribly nervous.

Tossing the velvet ribbon over her shoulder, she said to a woman standing by, "Is this Mrs Scott's house?"

And the woman, smiling queerly, said, "It is, my lass."

Oh, to be away from this! Laura actually said, "Help me, God," as she walked up the tiny path and knocked.

Then the door was opened by a little woman in black.

Laura said, "Are you Mrs Scott?"

But to her horror the woman answered, "Walk in please, miss," and Laura was shut in the passage.

"No," said Laura, "I don't want to come in. I only want to leave this basket. Mother sent—"

THE GARDEN PARTY

The little woman in the gloomy passage seemed not to have heard her. "Step this way, please, miss," she said in an oily voice, and Laura followed her.

She found herself in a wretched little low kitchen, lighted by a smoky lamp. There was another woman sitting before the fire.

"Em," said the little creature who had let her in. "Em! It's a young lady." She turned to Laura. "Em's Mrs Scott, miss. I'm 'er sister. You'll excuse 'er, won't you?" she said.

"Oh, but of course!" said Laura. "Please, please don't disturb her. I – I only want to leave – "

But at that moment the woman at the fire turned round. Her face, puffed up, red, with swollen eyes and swollen lips, looked terrible. She seemed as though she couldn't understand why Laura was there. What was it all about? And the poor face puckered up again.

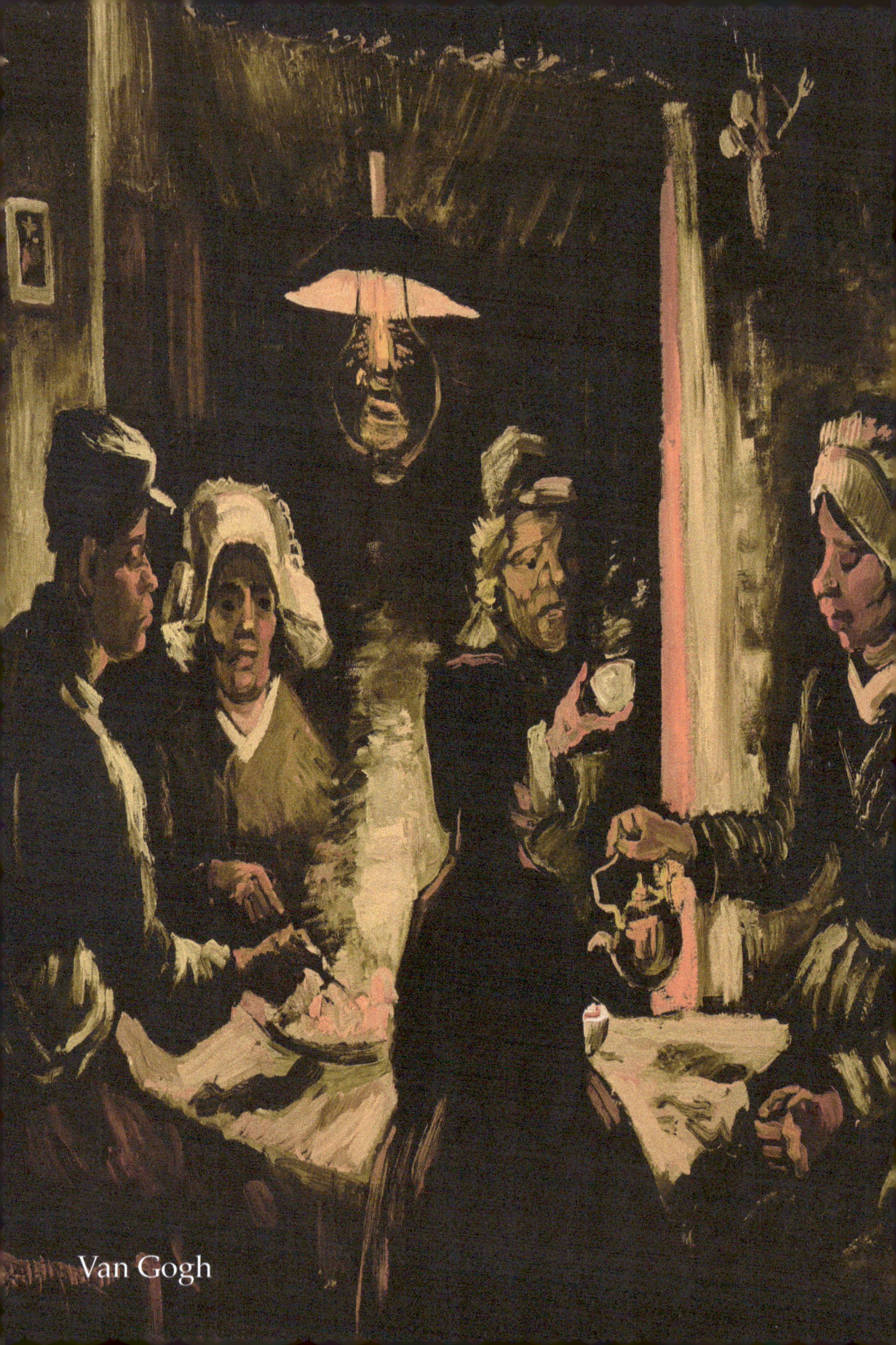
Van Gogh

"All right, my dear," said her sister. "I'll thenk the young lady."

And again she began, "You'll excuse her, m-miss, I'm sure," and her face, swollen too, tried an oily smile.

Laura only wanted to get out, to get away. She was back in the passage. A door opened, and accidentally she walked straight through into the bedroom, where the dead man was lying.

"You'd like a look at 'im, wouldn't you?" said Em's sister, and she brushed past Laura over to the bed. "'e looks a picture. There's nothing to show. Come along, my dear."

Laura came.

There lay a young man, fast asleep – sleeping so soundly, so deeply, that he was far, far away from them both. Oh, so remote, so peaceful. He was dreaming. His eyes were closed. He was given up to his dream.

What did garden parties and baskets and lace frocks matter to him? He was far from all those things. He was wonderful, beautiful. While they were laughing and while the band was playing, this marvel had come to the lane. Happy… happy… All is well, said that sleeping face. This is just as it should be. I am content.

But all the same you had to cry, and Laura couldn't go out of the room without saying something to him. She gave a sob.

"Forgive my hat," she said.

And this time she didn't wait for Em's sister. She found her way out of the door, down the path. At the corner of the lane she met Laurie.

He stepped out of the shadow. "Is that you, Laura? Mother was getting anxious. Was it all right?"

"Yes, quite. Oh, Laurie!" She took his arm, she pressed up against him.

"I say, you're not crying, are you?" asked her brother. He put his arm round her shoulder. "Don't cry," he said in his warm, loving voice. "Was it awful?"

"No," sobbed Laura. "It was simply marvellous. But Laurie – " She stopped, she looked at her brother. "Isn't life," she stammered, "isn't life – " But what life was she couldn't explain. No matter. He quite understood.

"Isn't it, darling?" said Laurie.

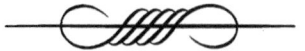

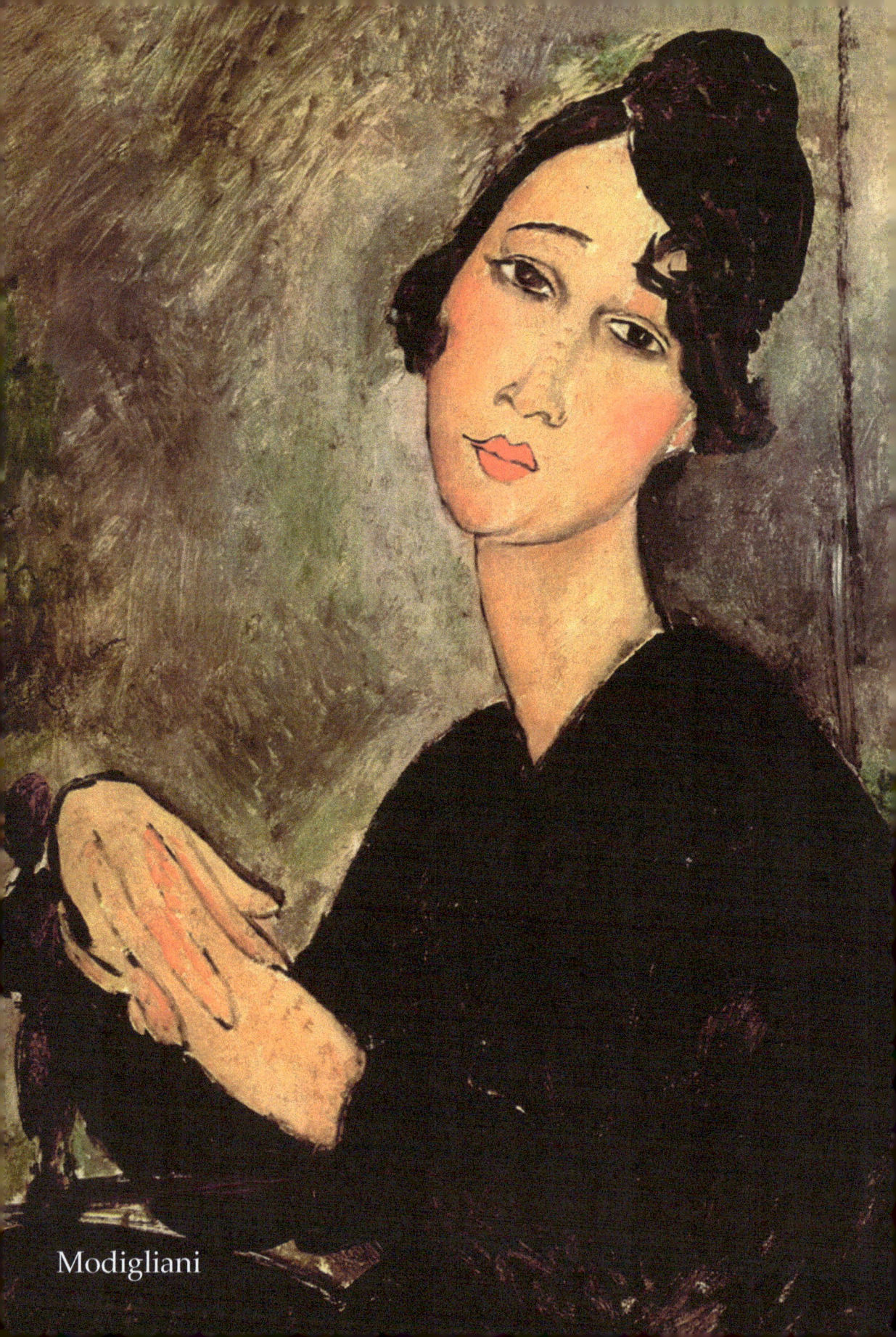

PRÉCIS OF THE STORY

The Sheridans are preparing to hold their annual garden party in their Wellington home. When daughters Laura and Jose Sheridan are helping with the preparations, they hear that a man from the poor cottages nearby has been killed in an accident with a cart.

Laura thinks the garden party ought to be cancelled to show respect to the dead man, but her mother tells her that "people like that don't expect sacrifices from us." The garden party is not cancelled, and is a great success.

However, afterwards, Mrs Sheridan, wishing to appear generous and sympathetic, sends Laura to the dead man's widow with a basket of food left over from the garden party. Laura is reluctant to go, but sees that the dead man is at peace. Laura marvels at his deep contentment.

THE DOLL'S HOUSE

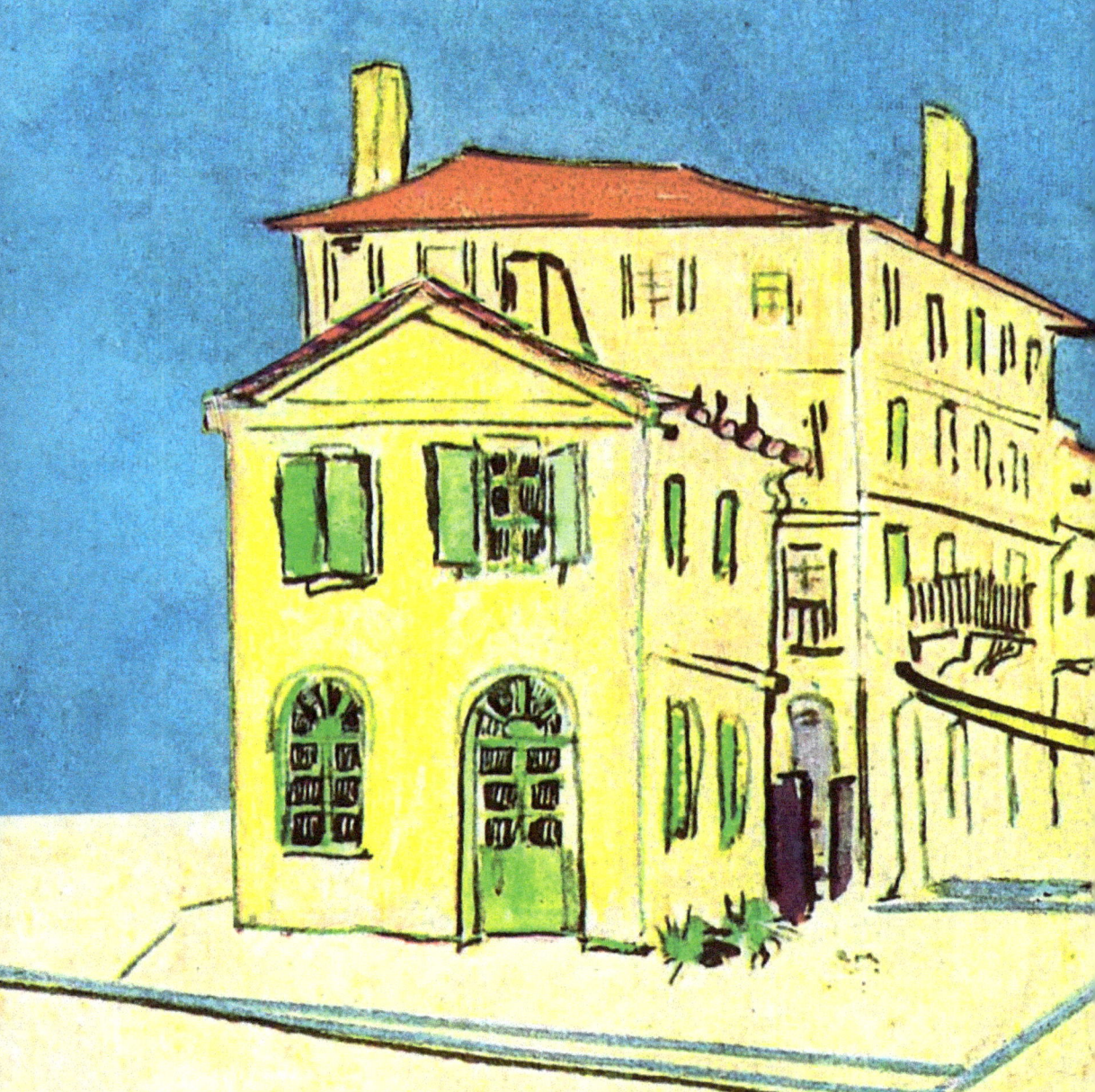

Illustration adapted from Van Gogh

CAST OF CHARACTERS

Isabel Burnell
Lottie Burnell } Owners of the Doll's House
Kezia Burnell

Mrs Burnell, mother of Isabel, Lottie and Kezia

Aunt Beryl, aunt of Isabel, Lottie and Kezia

Lil Kelvey } The Kelvey sisters
'Our Else' Kelvey

Mrs Kelvey, a washerwoman and mother of Lil and Our Else.

Lena Logan
Emmie Cole } School friends of Isabel, Lottie and Kezia
Jessie May

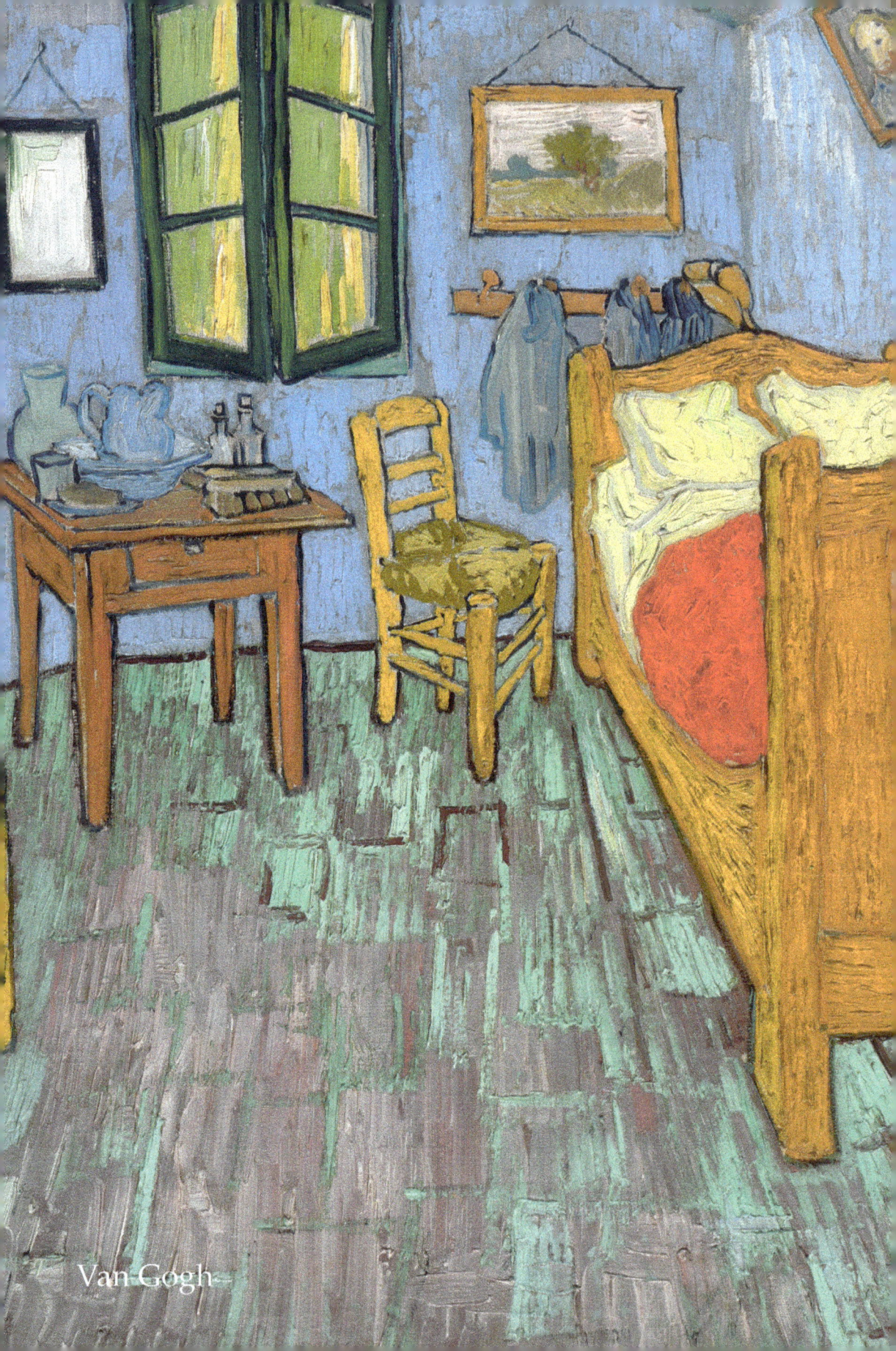

THE DOLL'S HOUSE

The Burnell children, Isabel, Lottie and Kezia, had been given a doll's house.

The doll's house was painted a dark, oily, spinach green, picked out with bright yellow. It was placed outside in the courtyard because it was so big, and because the smell of new paint was so strong.

Isabel, Lottie and Kezia Burnell thought the doll's house was too marvellous; it was too much for them.

The Burnell children had never seen anything like it in their lives. All the rooms were papered. There were pictures on the walls, painted on the paper, with gold frames complete.

Red carpet covered all the floors except the kitchen. Red plush chairs were in the drawing-room, green in the dining-room. There were tables, beds with real bedclothes, a cradle, a stove, a dresser with tiny plates and one big jug.

But what Kezia liked more than anything,
what she liked frightfully, was the lamp.
It stood in the middle of the dining-room
table, an exquisite little amber lamp with a
white globe.

The lamp was even filled all ready for
lighting, though, of course, you couldn't light
it. But there was something inside that looked
like oil, and that moved when you shook it.

The lamp was perfect. It seemed to smile to
Kezia, to say, "I live here." The lamp was real.

"I'm to tell," said Isabel, "because I'm
the eldest. And you two can join in after.
But I'm to tell first."

The Burnell children could hardly walk
to school fast enough the next morning.
They burned to tell everybody, to describe,
to – well – to boast about their doll's house
before the school-bell rang.

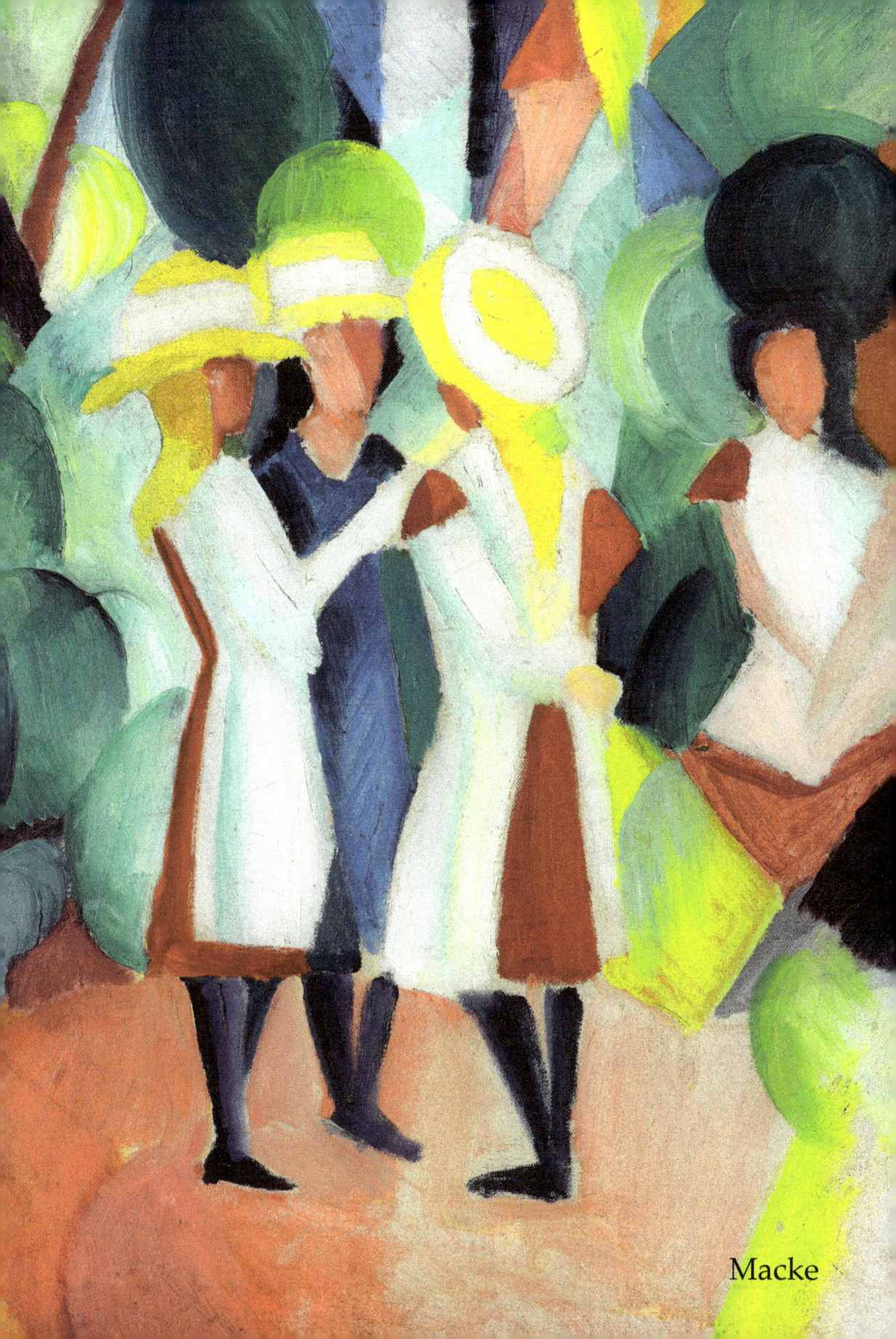

There was nothing to answer. Isabel was bossy, but she was always right, and Lottie and Kezia knew too well the powers that went with being eldest.

The Burnells' mother had arranged that while the doll's house stood in the courtyard they might ask the girls at school, two at a time, to come and look. Not to stay to tea, of course. But just to stand quietly in the courtyard while Isabel pointed out the beauties, and Lottie and Kezia looked pleased.

Isabel said: "And I'm to choose who's to come and see it first. Mother said I might."

But when Isabel, Lottie and Kezia reached school, they couldn't tell anyone immediately, because it was time for the roll to be called.

Never mind. Isabel tried to make up for it by looking very important and mysterious and by whispering behind her hand to the girls near her, "Got something to tell you at playtime."

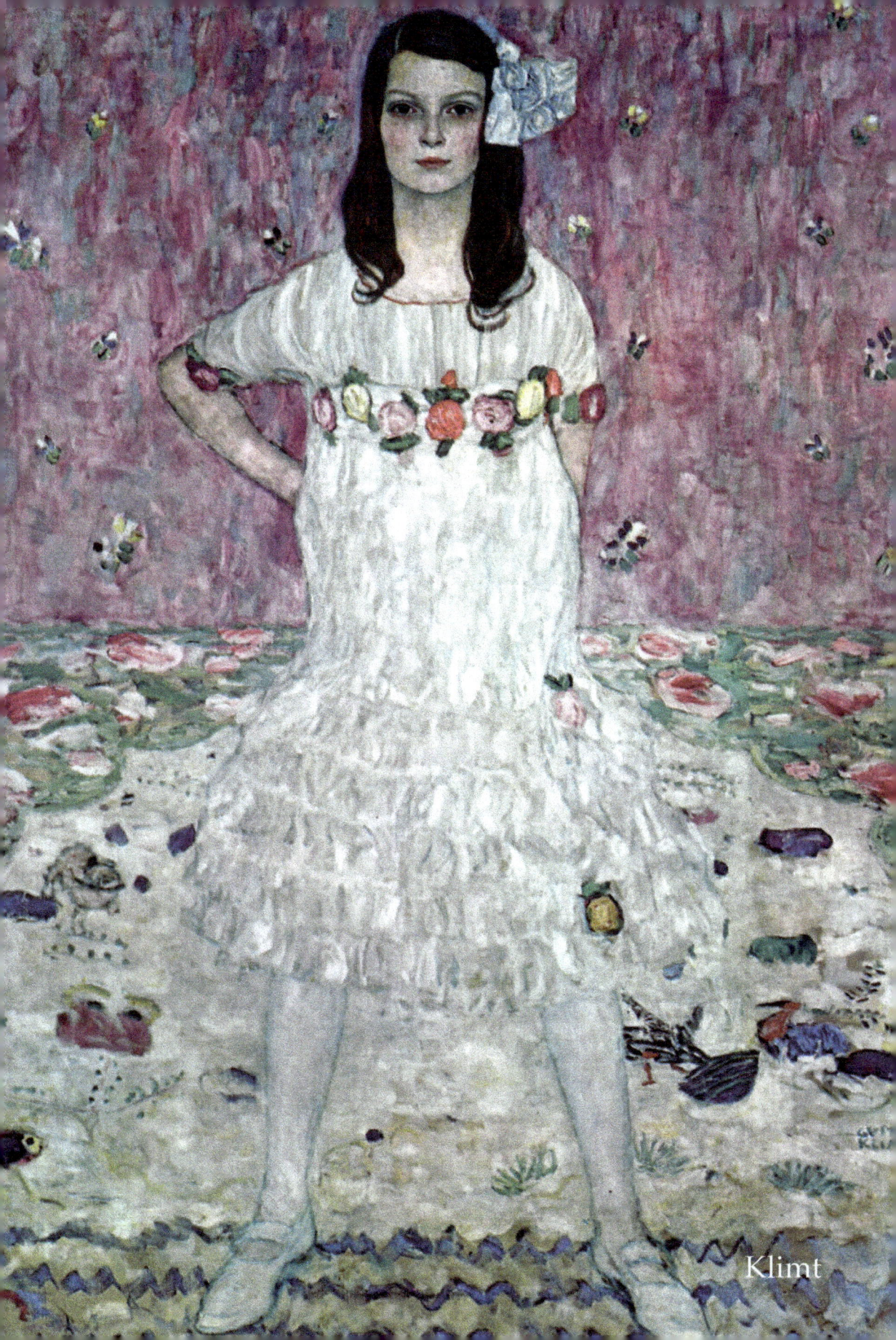

Playtime came and Isabel was surrounded.
The girls of her class nearly fought to put their
arms round her, to walk away with her, to
beam flatteringly, to be her special friend.

Only two children stayed outside the ring
of Isabel Burnell's special friends. These
were the two who were always outside,
the little Kelveys.

Many of the children, including the Burnells,
were not allowed even to speak to the
Kelveys. And as the Burnells set the fashion
in all matters of behaviour, the Kelveys were
shunned by everybody.

They were not the children of the judge,
the doctor, or even the store-keeper or
the milkman.

They were the daughters of a spry, hard-
working little washerwoman. This was awful
enough. But where was Mr Kelvey? Nobody
knew for certain. But everybody said he was
in prison.

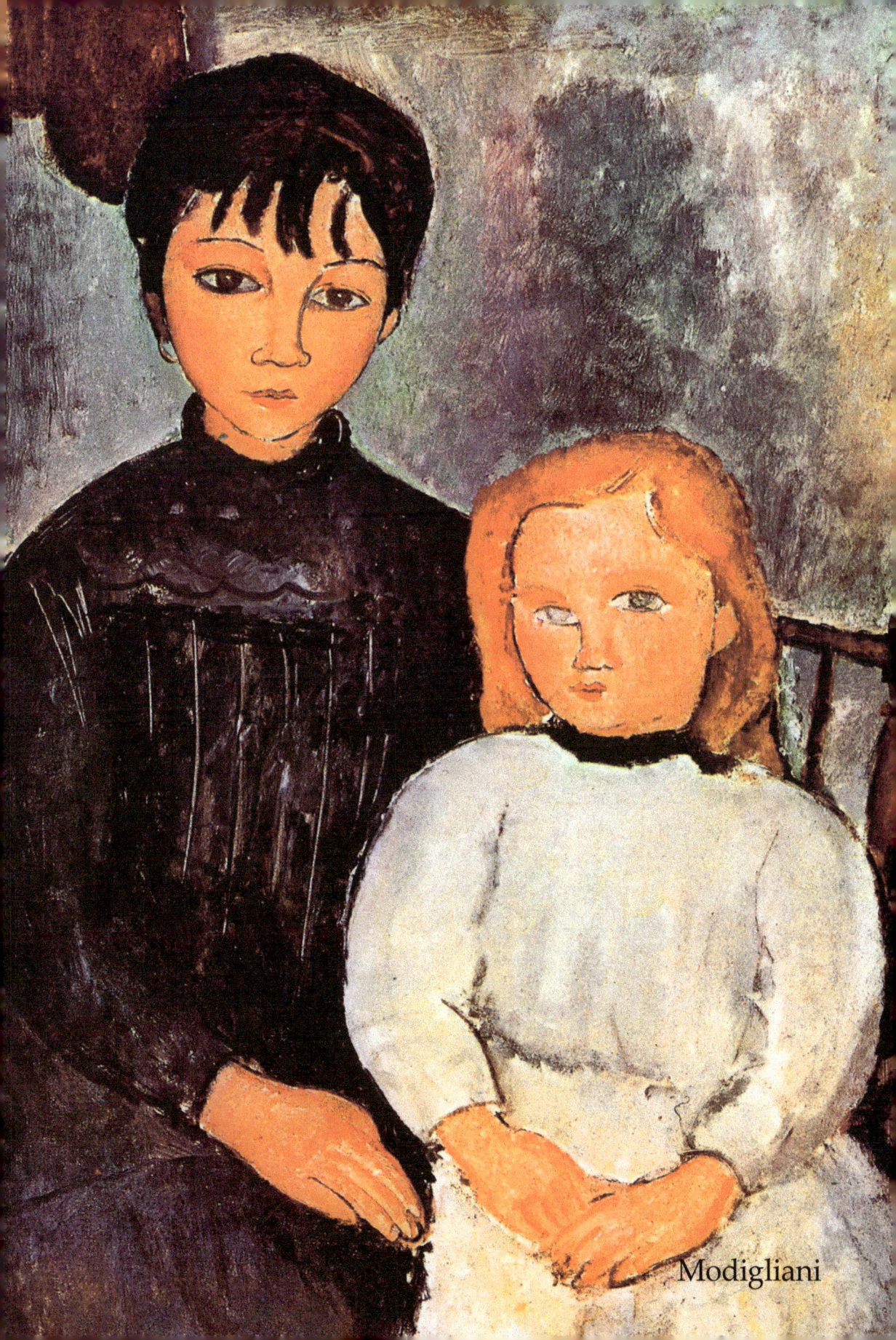

So the little Kelveys were the daughters of a washerwoman and a jailbird. Very nice company for other people's children!

And they looked it. Mrs Kelvey was obliged to dress them in "bits" given to her by the people for whom she worked. Lil, a stout, plain child, came to school in a dress made from a green art-serge table-cloth of the Burnells, with red plush sleeves from the Logans' curtains.

And her little sister, Our Else, wore a long white dress, rather like a nightgown, and a pair of little boy's boots. But whatever Our Else wore she would have looked strange. She was a tiny wishbone of a child, with cropped hair and enormous solemn eyes – a little white owl.

Our Else went through life holding on to Lil, with a piece of Lil's skirt screwed up in her hand. Where Lil went Our Else followed.

When she wanted anything, Our Else gave Lil a tug, a twitch, and Lil stopped and turned round. The Kelveys never failed to understand each other.

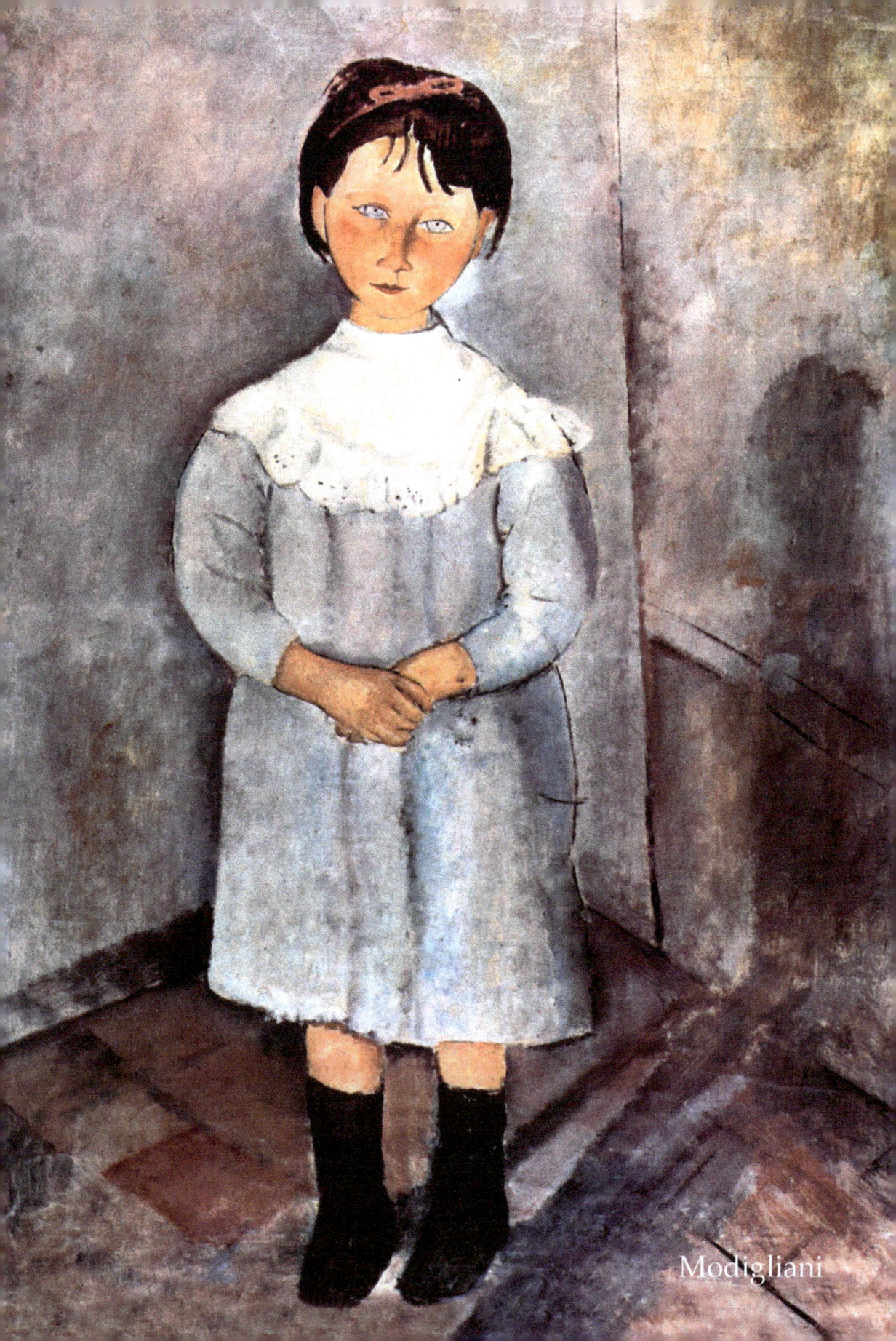

When Isabel talked about the doll's house, the little Kelveys hovered at the edge; you couldn't stop them listening. When the other little girls turned round and sneered, Lil, as usual, gave her silly, shame-faced smile, but Our Else only looked.

While the little Kelveys looked, Isabel went on telling, about the carpet, the beds with real bedclothes, and the stove with an oven door.

When she finished Kezia broke in. "You've forgotten the lamp, Isabel."

"Oh, yes," said Isabel, "and there's a teeny little lamp, all made of yellow glass, with a white globe that stands on the dining-room table. You couldn't tell it from a real one."

"The lamp's best of all," cried Kezia. She thought Isabel wasn't making half enough of the little lamp.

THE DOLL'S HOUSE

When the school girls knew they were all to have a chance to view the doll's house, they couldn't be nice enough to Isabel. One by one they put their arms round Isabel's waist, saying, "Isabel's my friend."

Only the little Kelveys moved away forgotten; there was nothing more for them to hear.

Days passed, and as more children saw the doll's house, the fame of it spread. It became the one subject, the rage. The one question was, "Have you seen Burnells' doll's house?" "Oh, ain't it lovely!"

Even during the dinner hour everyone was talking about the doll's house. The school girls sat under the pines eating their thick mutton sandwiches and big slabs of johnny cake spread with butter.

While always, as near as they could get, sat the Kelveys, Our Else holding on to Lil, listening too, while they chewed their jam sandwiches out of a newspaper soaked with large red blobs.

"Mother," said Kezia, "can't I ask the Kelveys just once?"

"Certainly not, Kezia."

"But why not?"

"Run away, Kezia; you know quite well why not."

At last everybody had seen the doll's house except the Kelveys.

It was the dinner hour. The children stood together under the pine trees, and suddenly, as they looked at the Kelveys eating out of their paper, always by themselves, always listening, they wanted to be horrid to them.

Emmie Cole started the whisper. "Lil Kelvey's going to be a servant when she grows up."

"O-oh, how awful!" said Isabel Burnell.

Then Lena Logan's little eyes snapped.

"Shall I ask her?" she whispered.

"Bet you don't," said Jessie May.

"Pooh. I'm not frightened," said Lena.

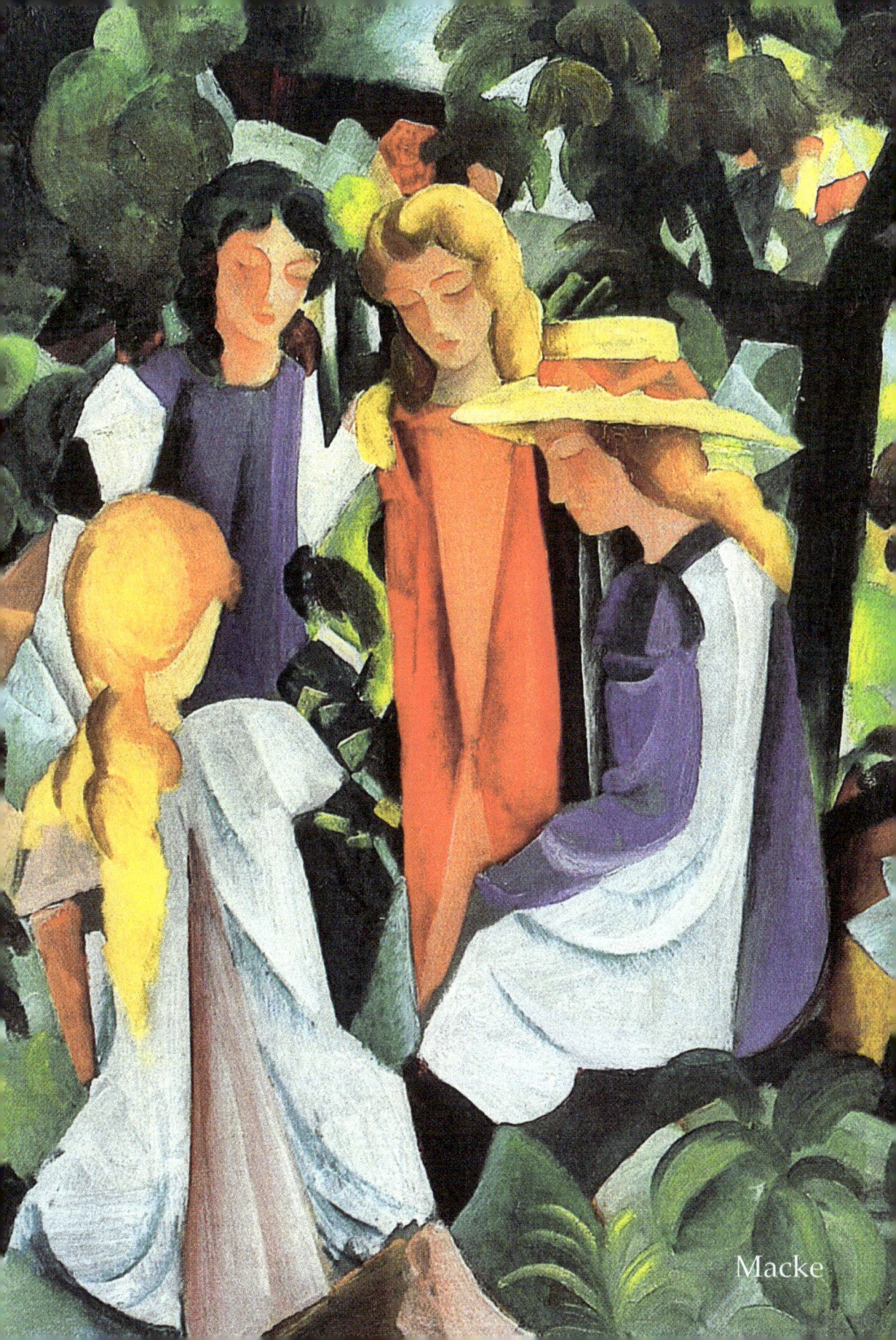

Giggling behind her hand, Lena went over to the Kelveys. Lil looked up from her dinner. Our Else stopped chewing. What was coming now?

"Is it true you're going to be a servant when you grow up, Lil Kelvey?" shrilled Lena.

Dead silence. Instead of answering, Lil only gave her silly, shame-faced smile. She didn't seem to mind the question at all. What a sell for Lena! The girls began to titter.

Lena couldn't stand that. She put her hands on her hips; she shot forward. "Yah, yer father's in prison!" she hissed, spitefully.

This was such a marvellous thing to have said that Lena, Jessie and Emmie as well as the Burnell girls rushed away in a body, deeply, deeply excited, wild with joy.

In the afternoon, the Burnell children had visitors, and Isabel and Lottie went upstairs to change their pinafores.

But Kezia thieved out at the back. She saw the little Kelveys coming up the road. Kezia hesitated. The Kelveys came nearer, and beside them walked their shadows, very long, stretching right across the road with their heads in the buttercups.

Kezia made up her mind. "Hullo," she said to the passing Kelveys. The Kelvey girls were so astounded that they stopped. Lil gave her silly smile. Our Else stared.

"You can come and see our doll's house if you want to," said Kezia to the little Kelveys, and she dragged one toe on the ground. But at that Lil turned red and shook her head quickly.

"Why not?" asked Kezia.

Lil gasped, then she said, "Your ma told our ma you wasn't to speak to us."

"Oh, well," said Kezia. She didn't know what to reply. "It doesn't matter. You can come and see our doll's house all the same. Come on. Nobody's looking."

But Lil shook her head still harder.

"Don't you want to?" asked Kezia.

Suddenly there was a twitch, a tug at Lil Kelvey's skirt. She turned round. Our Else was looking at her with big, imploring eyes; she was frowning. She wanted to see the doll's house.

Lil started forward. Kezia led the way. Like two little stray cats Lil and Our Else followed across the courtyard to where the doll's house stood.

"There it is," said Kezia.

There was a pause. Lil breathed loudly, almost snorted; Our Else was still as a stone.

"I'll open it for you," said Kezia kindly. She undid the hook and they looked inside.

"There's the drawing-room and the dining-room, and that's the…"

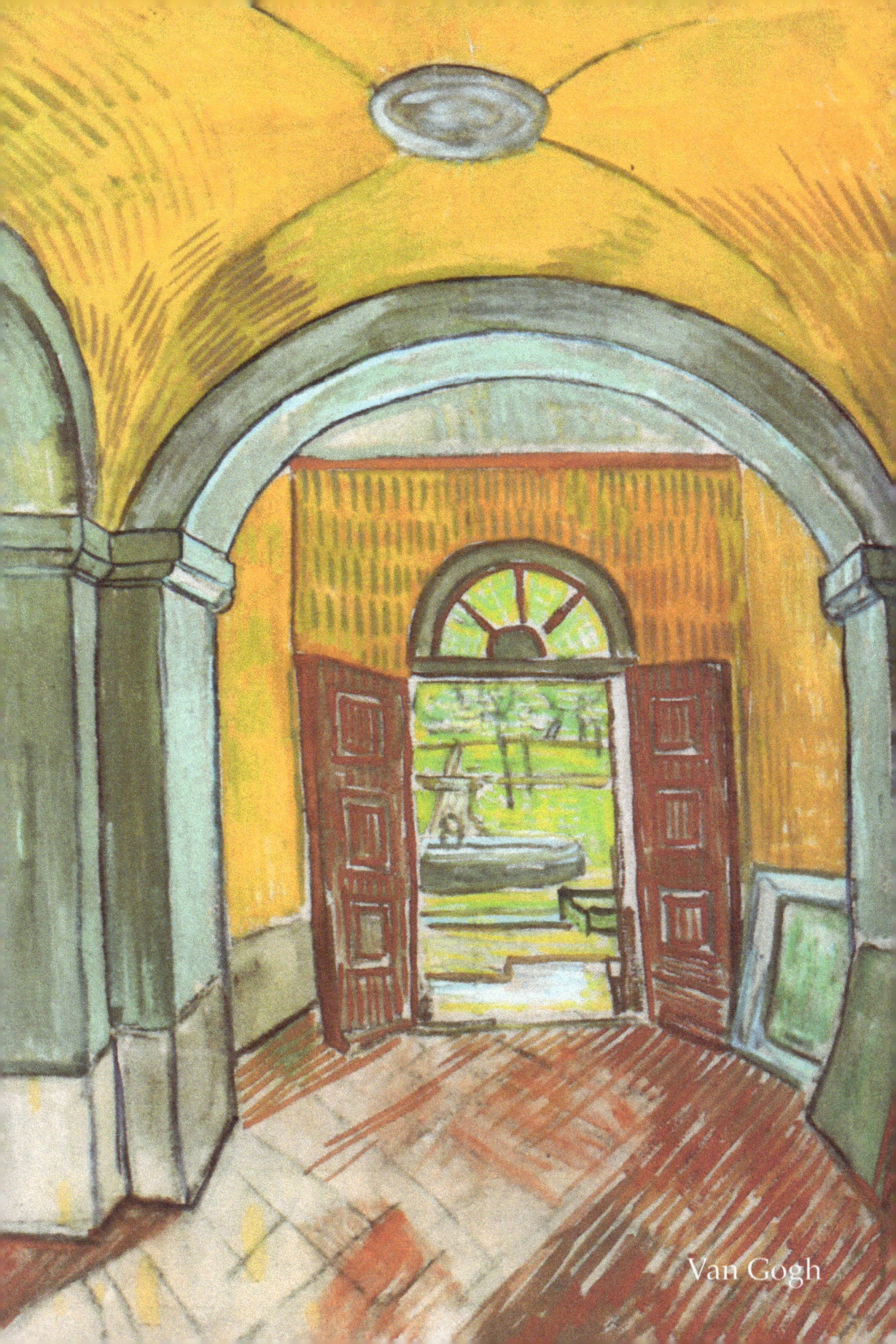

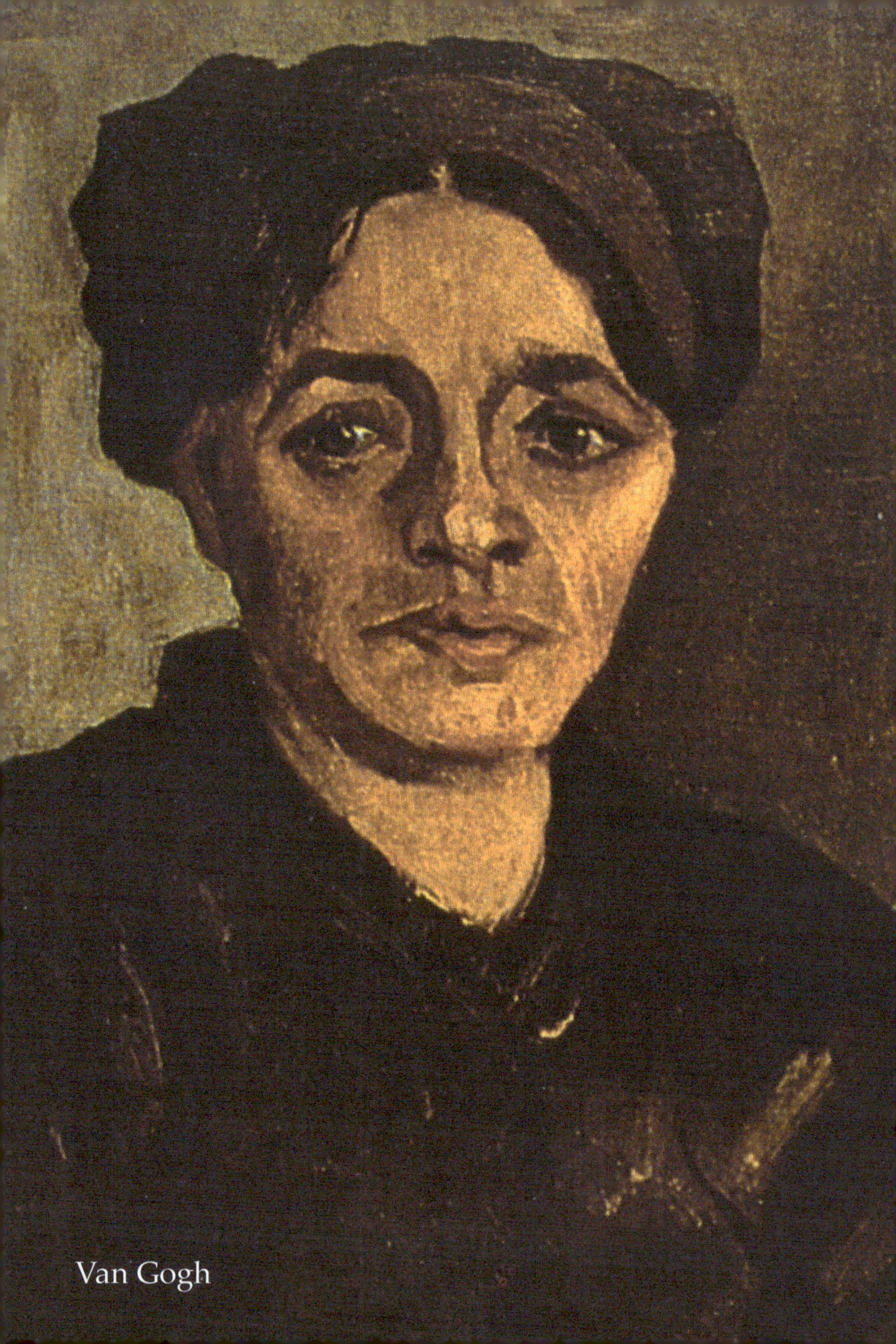
Van Gogh

THE DOLL'S HOUSE

"Kezia!" Oh, what a start they gave! "Kezia!" It was Aunt Beryl's voice.

At the back door stood the Burnell children's Aunt Beryl, staring as if she couldn't believe what she saw.

"How dare you ask the little Kelveys into the courtyard?" said her cold, furious voice. "You know as well as I do, you're not allowed to talk to them." And she stepped into the yard and shooed them out as if they were chickens.

"Off you go immediately!" she called, cold and proud.

Lil and Our Else did not need telling twice. Burning with shame, shrinking together, somehow they crossed the big courtyard and squeezed through the white gate.

When the Kelveys were well out of sight of Burnells', they sat down to rest on a big red drain-pipe by the side of the road. Lil's cheeks were still burning.

Dreamily they looked over the hay paddocks, past the creek, to the group of wattles where Logan's cows stood waiting to be milked. What were their thoughts?

Presently Our Else nudged up close to her sister. But now she had forgotten the cross lady. She smiled her rare smile.

"I seen the little lamp," she said, softly.

Then both were silent once more.

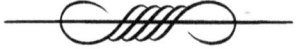

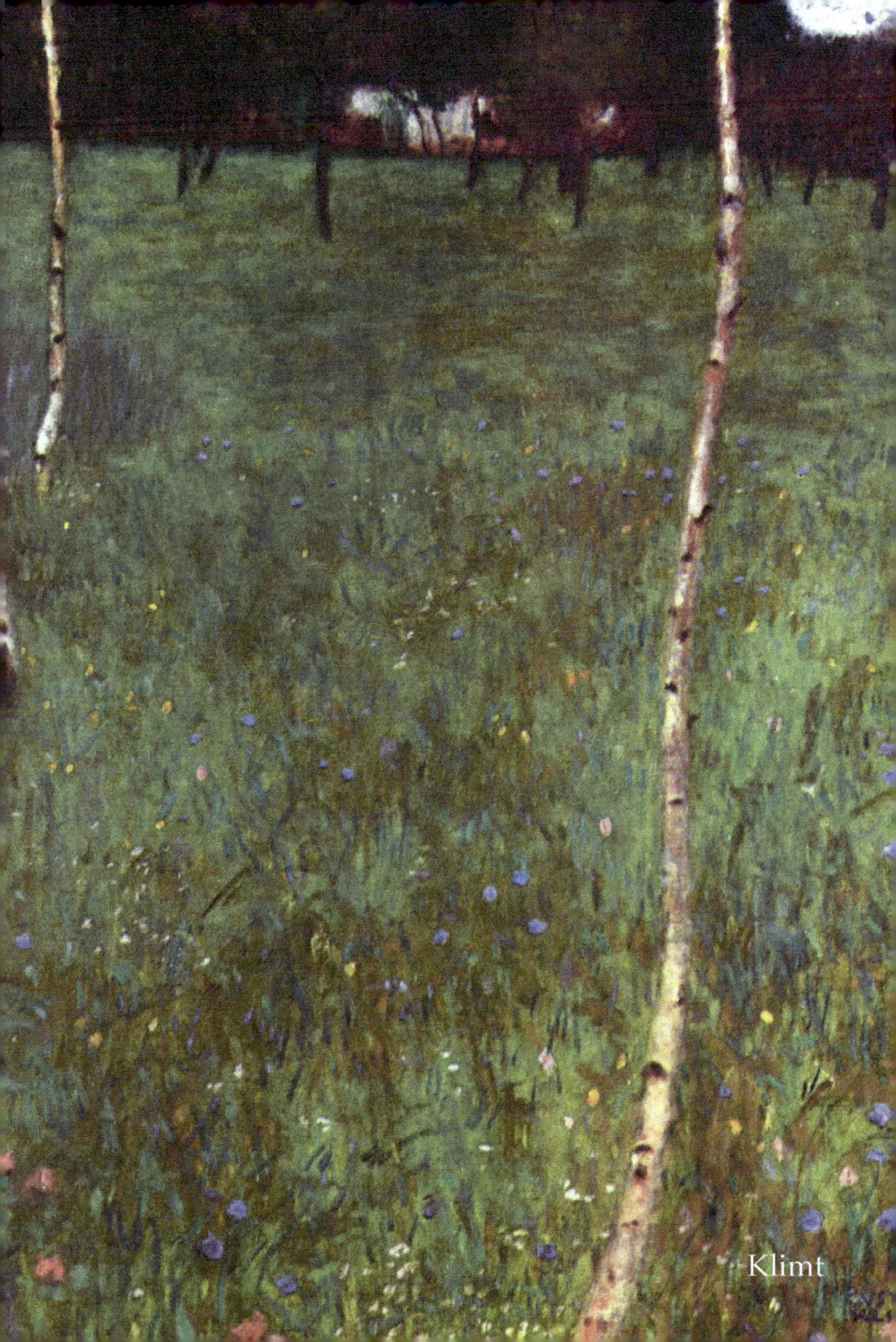

PRÉCIS OF THE STORY

The Burnell sisters, Isabel, Lottie and Kezia, are given a doll's house, and they proudly tell their friends about it at school. Kezia thinks the very best thing in it is a tiny oil lamp, which looks as if it has real oil in it.

Nearly all the schoolgirls are invited to look at the doll's house, except the little Kelvey sisters. Lil and Our Else Kelvey are dressed in hand-me-down clothes. Their mother is a washerwoman, and father is rumoured to be in jail.

Kezia takes pity on the little Kelveys, and asks them into the courtyard to view the doll's house. But the Burnells' Aunt Beryl catches Lil and Our Else and shoos them away as if they were chickens. The Kelvey sisters are mortified, but afterwards, they forget about the angry aunt, and are happy that they too have seen "the little lamp."

ABOUT KATHERINE MANSFIELD

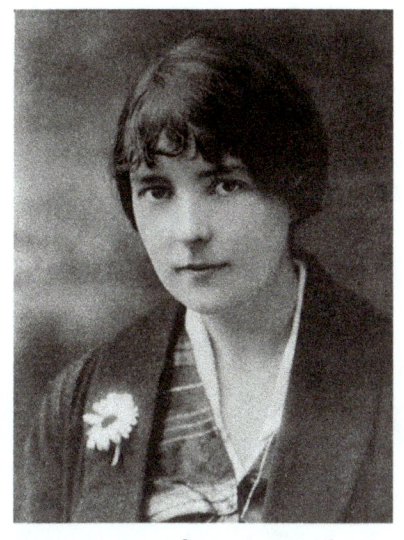

Katherine Mansfield was born in 1888 in Wellington, New Zealand, into a socially prominent family. She went to secondary school in London and returned back to New Zealand three years later, in 1906, to write stories. She returned to London in 1908 to focus on becoming a professional writer. In Europe, her circle of friends included Virginia Woolf and D. H. Lawrence. She contracted tuberculosis but still continued to publish acclaimed collections, such as *The Garden Party* and *Bliss*. Sadly, this great talent died of tuberculosis in 1923, aged 34.

The Katherine Mansfield Birthplace, in Wellington, New Zealand, open to the public, celebrates the life of New Zealand's most famous author.

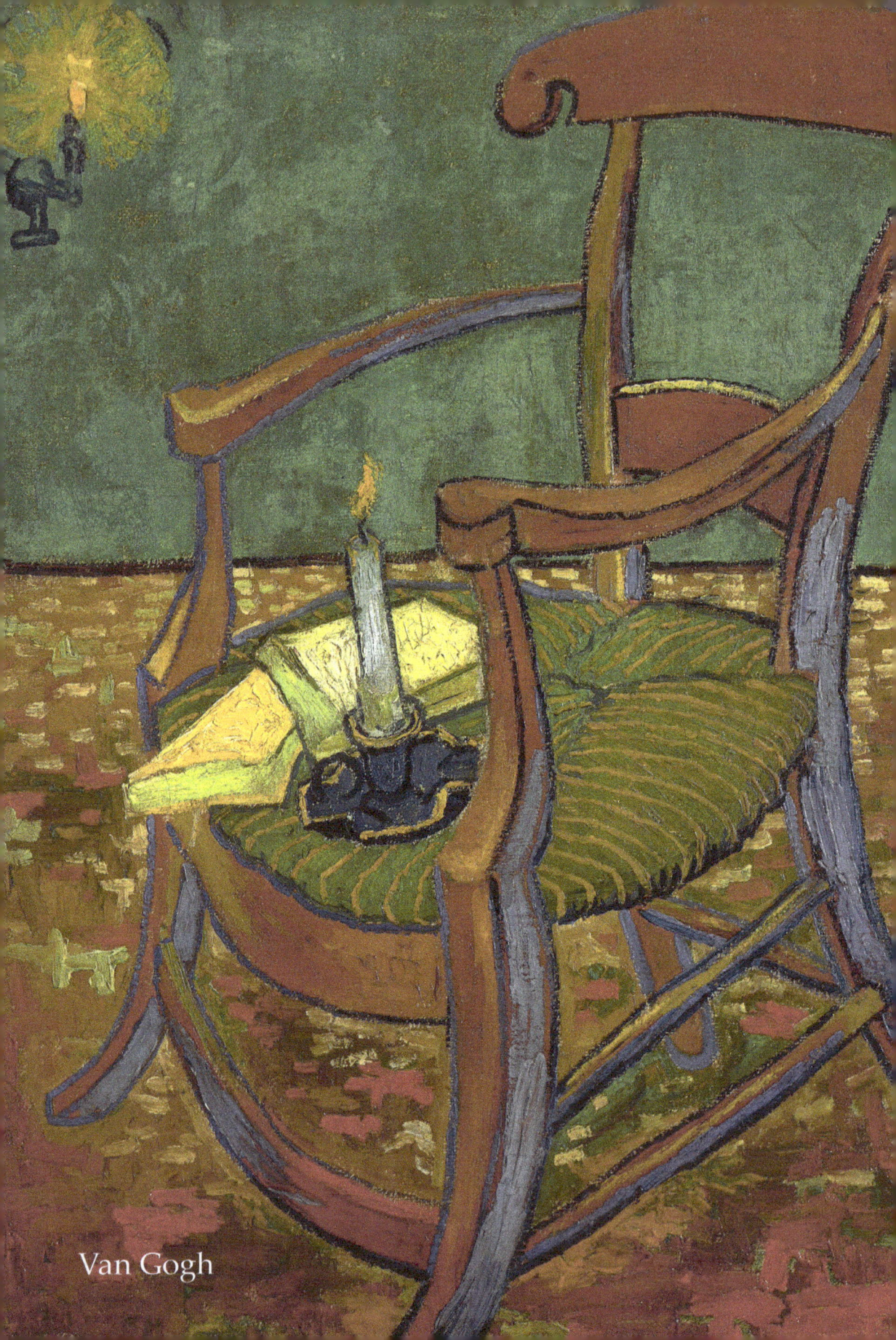
Van Gogh

www.ingramcontent.com/pod-product-compliance
Lightning Source LLC
Chambersburg PA
CBHW051618030426
42334CB00030B/3238